Mediterranean Diet Cookbook for Beginners 2022

1000 Days Easy and Healthy Mediterranean Recipes with 21 Days Meal Plan and A Beginner's Guide for Your Whole Family to Enjoy A New Lifestyle

Janette Farmer

Copyright© 2021By Janette FarmerAll Rights Reserved

This book is copyright protected. It is only for personal use. You cannot amend, distribute, sell, use, quote or paraphrase any part of the content within this book, without the consent of the author or publisher.

Under no circumstances will any blame or legal responsibility be held against the publisher, or author, for any damages, reparation, or monetary loss due to the information contained within this book, either directly or indirectly.

Disclaimer Notice:

Please note the information contained within this document is for educational and entertainment purposes only. All effort has been executed to present accurate, up to date, reliable, complete information. No warranties of any kind are declared or implied. Readers acknowledge that the author is not engaged in the rendering of legal, financial, medical or professional advice. The content within this book has been derived from various sources. Please consult a licensed professional before attempting any techniques outlined in this book.

By reading this document, the reader agrees that under no circumstances is the author responsible for any losses, direct or indirect, that are incurred as a result of the use of the information contained within this document, including, but not limited to, errors, omissions, or inaccuracies.

CONTENT

Introduction 1

Chapter 1 Basics 16

Chapter 2 Beans and Grains 20

Chapter 3 Beef, Pork, and Lamb 30

Chapter 4 Breakfasts 40

Chapter 5 Desserts 50

Chapter 6 Fish and Seafood 61

Chapter 7 Meatless Mains 72

Chapter 8 Pizzas, Wraps, and Sandwiches 77

Chapter 9 Poultry 83

Chapter 10 Salads 89

Chapter 11 Snacks and Appetizers 100

Chapter 12 Staples, Sauces, Dips, and Dressings 110

Chapter 13 Stews and Soups 117

Chapter 14 Vegetables and Sides 126

Appendix 1 Measurement Conversion Chart 134

Appendix 2 The Dirty Dozen and Clean Fifteen 135

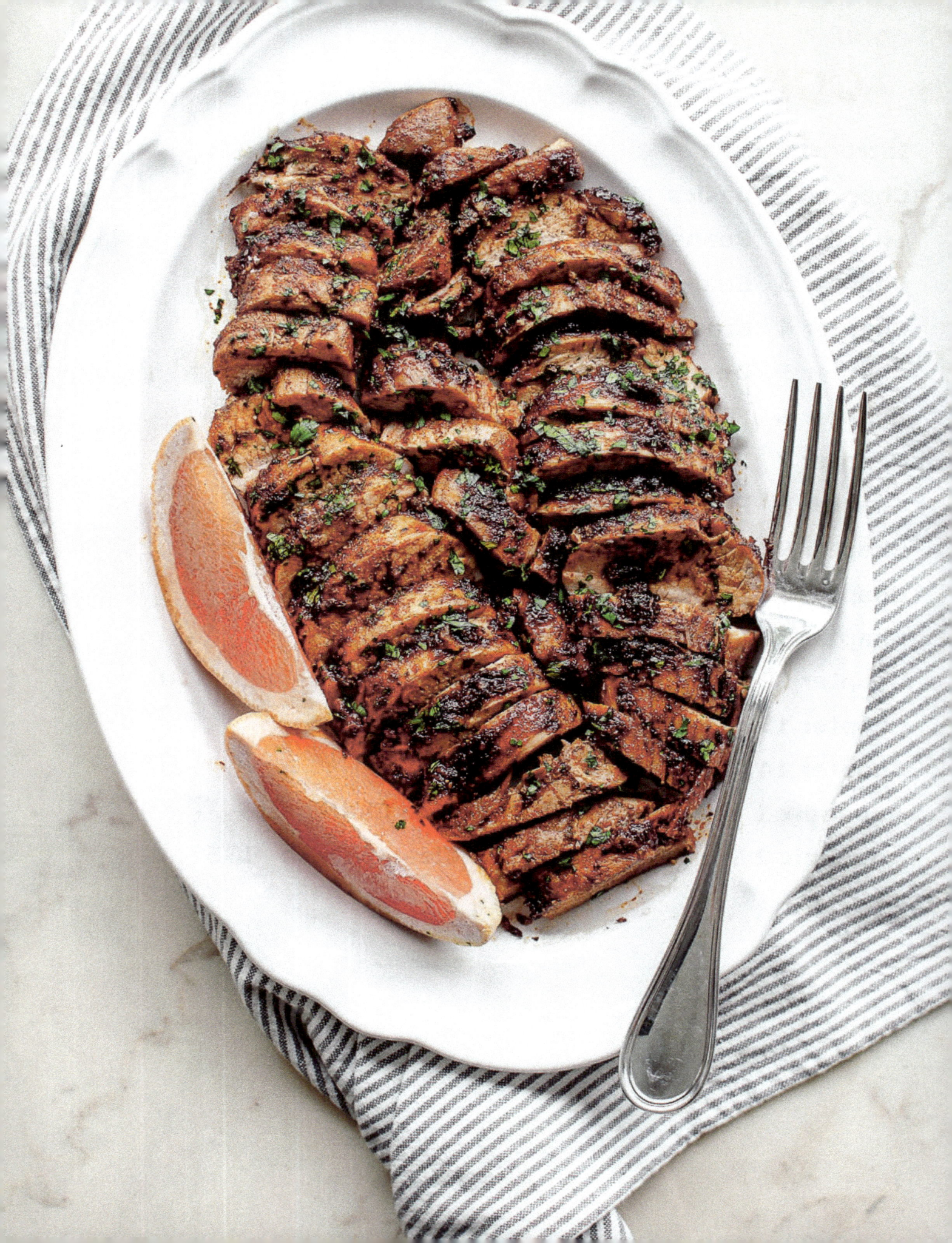

Introduction

The Mediterranean diet is gaining popularity amongst diet enthusiasts across the globe for the very right reasons. It has vast and significant medical and health benefits which are considered one of the major reasons for its widespread popularity. The diet is not restricting at all, and does not forbid you any food group from the food pyramid. You will get ample amount of nutritional foods on the Mediterranean diet, and that is why it is easier to adapt and stick to it. The Mediterranean diet is very promising in weight loss, and does not bound you to count calories for an effective weight loss approach. The diet lets you experience food in its natural flavors. This cookbook will act as your guide into understanding the Mediterranean diet, the foods you can eat and the restricted categories. This cookbook will also let you understand the vast medical benefits of the diet and the reason for why you should not waste a second to switch towards a happy and healthy lifestyle by following this amazing diet.

What Is the Mediterranean Diet?

Unlike some diets, the Mediterranean diet is relatively easy to adopt. This is because it is not too restrictive. This diet is based on the traditional diet of people who live around the Mediterranean sea, like from Italy, Spain, Greece, and Croatia. It is a diet that people naturally survived on and enjoyed. Therefore, it is not restrictive in the sense it follows an eating plan that people have lived on. Unlike some diets that people create, this diet has stood the test of time. It can easily be seen as a change in eating lifestyle. Rather than a strict meal plan, it's a way of eating that emphasizes fruits, vegetables, whole grains, legumes and olive oil. Fish is the main protein source instead of red meat, pork or poultry. And yes, it includes red wine in moderation. Fermented dairy is consumed regularly but in moderate amounts. Eggs and poultry are occasionally consumed, but red meat and sweets are not eaten regularly. It has been recommended by dieticians for improving heart health as it is plant-based and rich in healthy fats like olive oil and omega-3 fatty acids from fish. With this diet, the more colorful your plate looks, the better.

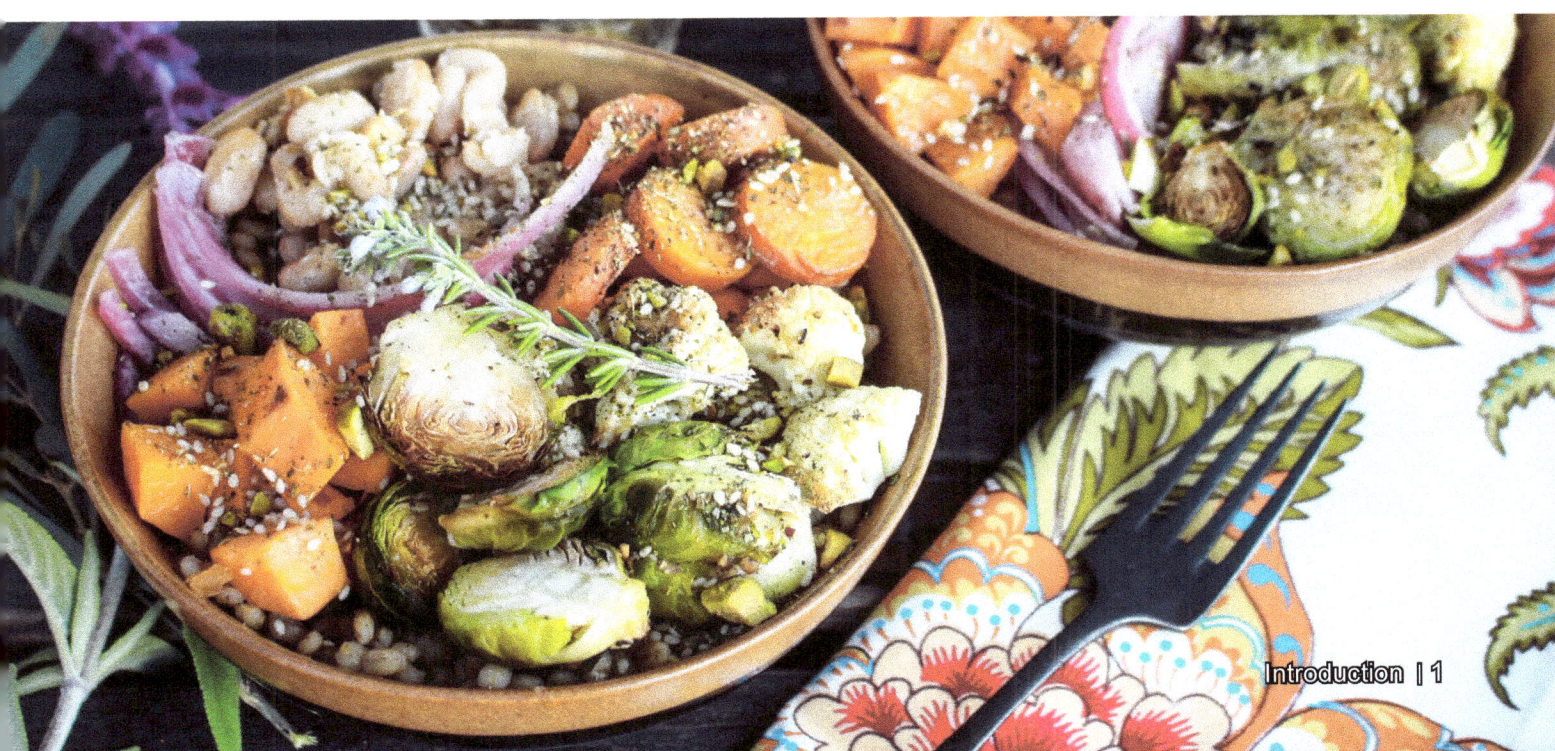

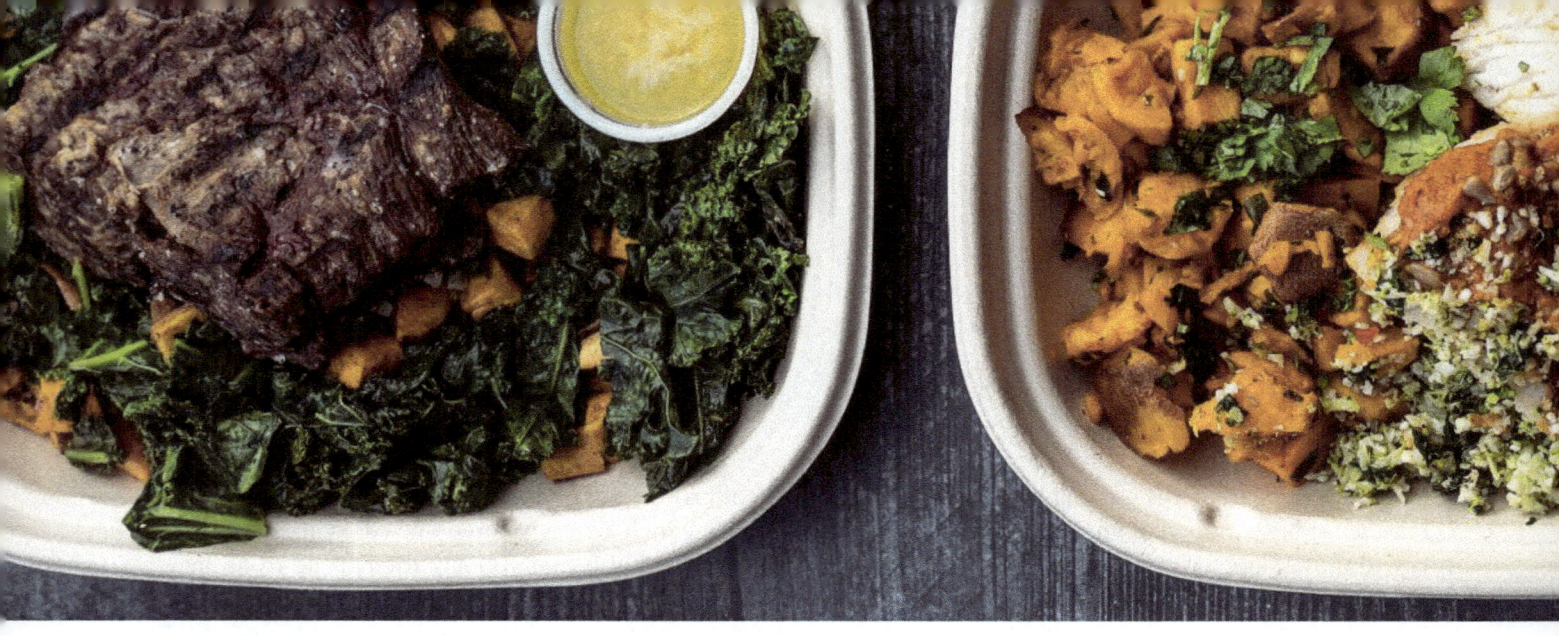

The Mediterranean Diet Pyramid

The Mediterranean diet was a result of the focus of the study conducted by Dr. Ancel Keys, known as the "Seven Countries Study", in light of epidemiology studies. Similarly, his research was backed by the WHO in the 1990s, stating that the people in the Mediterranean region were prone to a considerably lower risk of cardiovascular complications. The diet gain popularity when Dr. Walter Willett, i.e., HoD of the Nutrition Department at Harvard University, recommended it to a group of people. At that time, low-fat based diet plans were already recommended to people having cardiac issues. It was Dr. Willett who collaborated with the WHO to make the Mediterranean a renowned idea across the globe. His idea further evolved into the publishing of a diet pyramid based on various tiers and blocks somewhat similar to the USDA diet pyramid. The Mediterranean diet pyramid was primarily based on the Mediterranean diet plan and provided a systematic approach towards the diet plan.

The Mediterranean diet pyramid is basically a food pyramid that explains the most subtle and effective approach towards following the diet plan. The pyramid works as a guideline in understanding the ethos and the components of the diet plan in a more systematic and understandable manner. The Mediterranean diet pyramid was developed by Oldways, i.e., a Nutrition and Food Non-Profit Organization, in 1993 with the assistance and help of the World Health Organization and Harvard School of Public Health.

Categorically the first element or the base of the Mediterranean diet pyramid includes foods that are to be consumed every day. The foods at the bottom of the Mediterranean diet pyramid have to be included in almost all the daily meals. These foods include veggies, legumes, seeds, fruits, seeds, and olive oil. The base of the Mediterranean diet pyramid builds a systematic initial basis for adopting the diet plan as a necessary part of your food habits and inculcate a sense of healthiness.

The next step of the Mediterranean diet pyramid includes foods categories like seafood and fish. These foods have to be consumed a minimum of twice every week to have an effective and empowering Mediterranean diet plan in action. The third tier of the Mediterranean diet pyramid consists of foods that have to be consumed in a considerably reasonable manner ranging from daily to weekly basis. These food categories include poultry, yogurt, cheese, eggs, and in some instances, red wine. The

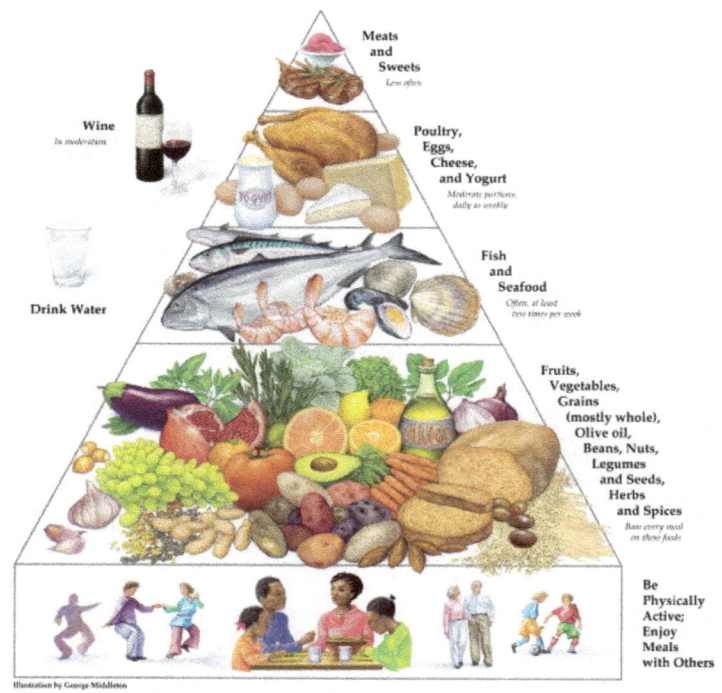

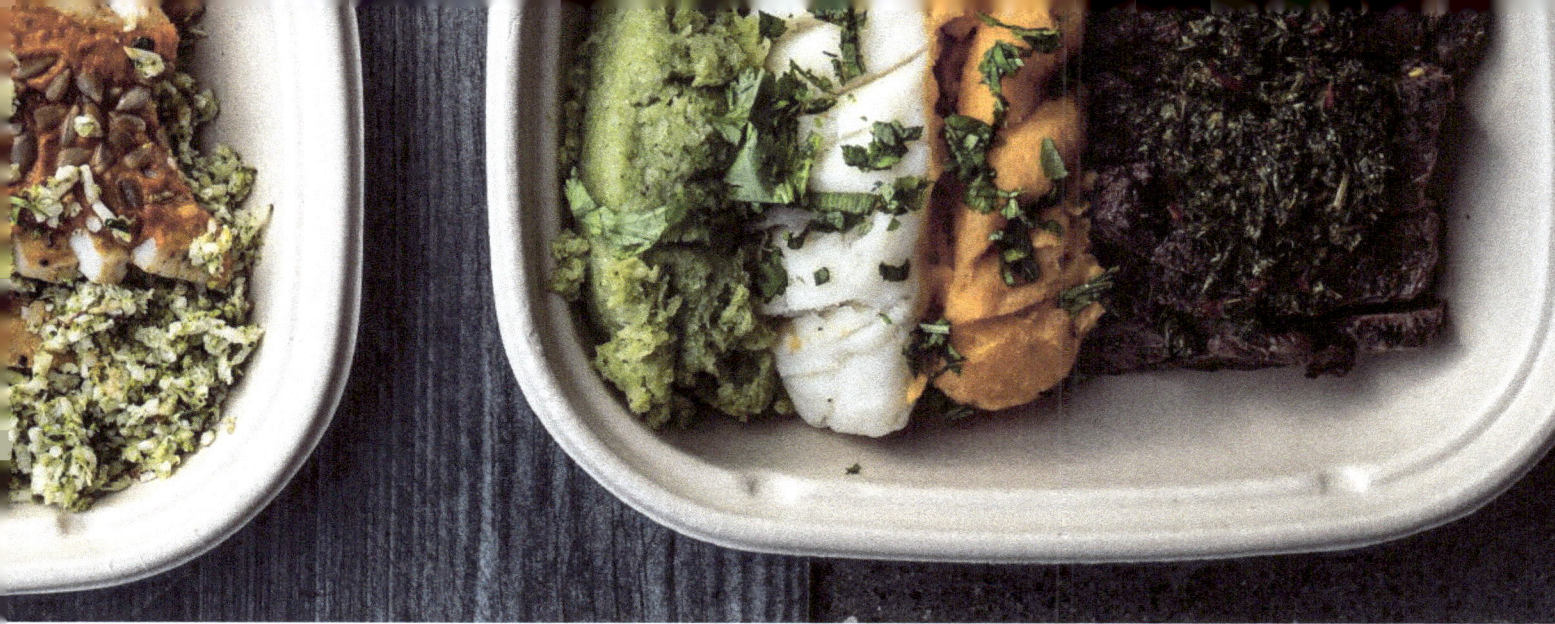

final or top tier of the Mediterranean diet pyramid consists of foods that have to be consumed less frequently or usually on special occasions. These food categories include saturated fats, red meat, and some sweet dishes.

One of the most important blocks of the Mediterranean diet pyramid is the exercise and physical workout. The Mediterranean diet pyramid also incorporates eating with others as an essential factor in living a healthy and nutritious lifestyle. It is imperative to thoroughly inculcate these two habits while following the Mediterranean diet. It is crucial to understand that a good diet cannot provide you with the benefits of a proper workout. Likewise, work out session cannot provide the benefits of a good diet. Therefore, having a combo of both a good diet and an effective workout plan is considered a key to a healthy lifestyle. Furthermore, food sharing is regarded as one of the most harmonious and oldest activities of human life. It has known to be effective in building solid relationships amongst fellow beings.

Before the Mediterranean diet pyramid was published, the USDA or United States Department of Agriculture had published their own diet pyramid model a year earlier. The peculiar factors in the USDA Diet Pyramid are as follows:
- The initial tier or base consists of 6 to 11 servings of carbs, including cereal, rice, bread, and pasta.
- The second block consists of 2 to 4 servings of fruits and 3 to 5 servings of veggies.
- The third block contains 2 to 3 servings of protein intake, including nuts, eggs, meat, fish, poultry, and beans. It also includes 2 to 3 servings of dairy products, including cheese, yogurt, and milk.
- The topmost tier of the USDA Diet Pyramid contains a moderate intake of sweets, fats, and oils.

The USDA Diet Pyramid is classified by category, and its daily recommended food consumption makes it considerably less flexible than the Mediterranean diet pyramid. It also provides a very limited approach towards the nutritional contribution of various foods. For example, veggies give a sufficient supply of fibre and carbs, and legumes offer both proteins and carbs.

The peculiar aspect of the Mediterranean diet pyramid is that it understands the differences between the nutritional outputs of the foods categorized as protein in the USDA diet pyramid. These food categories include meats, seafood, fish, dairy, and poultry. This difference in nutritional value explains how these foods should be used in meals effectively to maintain a healthy approach in eating habits.

Likewise, all the fats are categorized in one category in the USDA diet pyramid does not

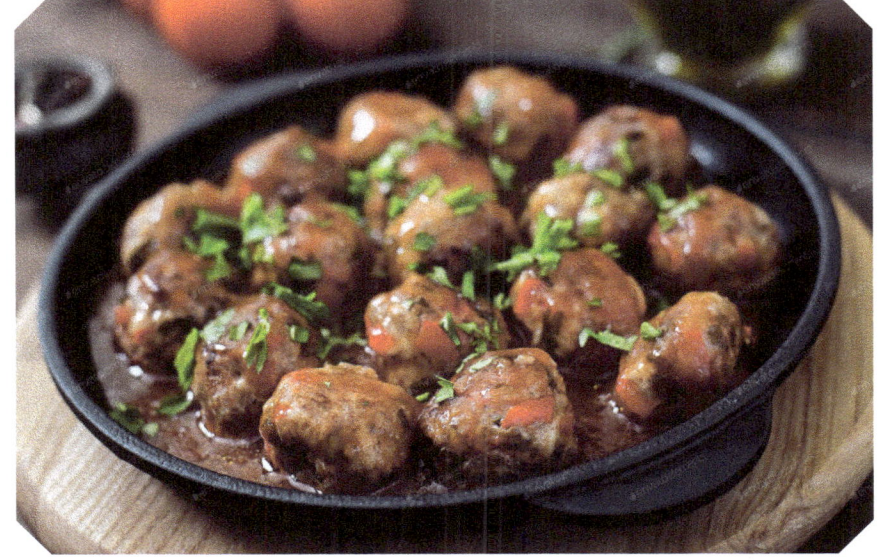

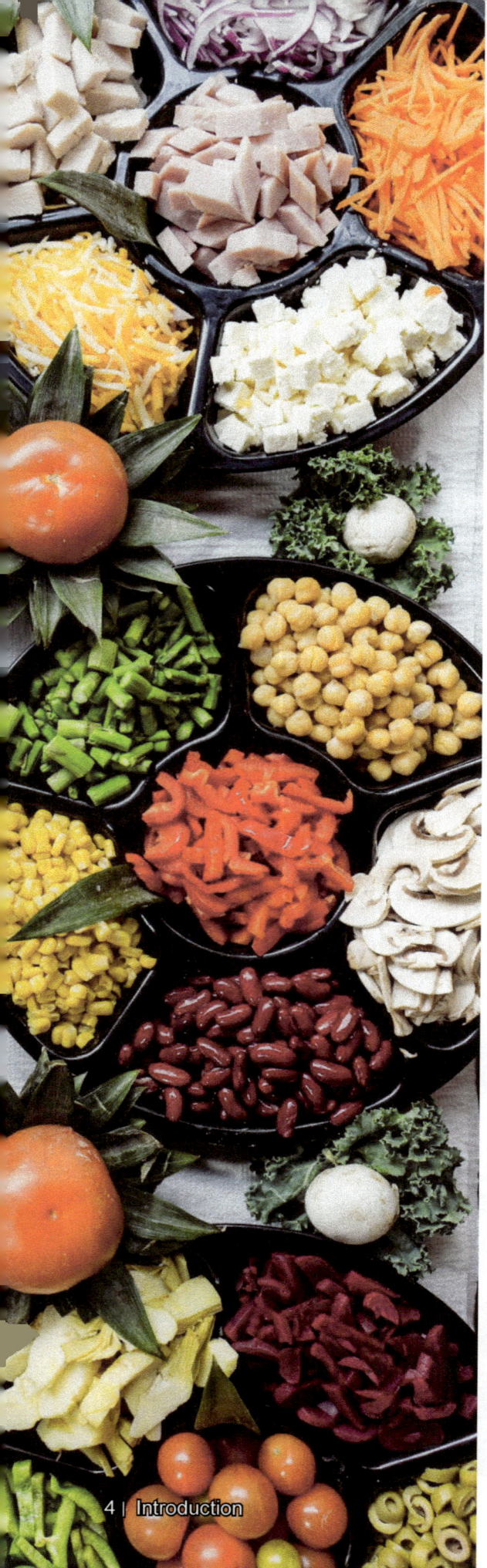

differentiate healthy fats like oils, seeds, and nuts, from trans fats and unsaturated fats. The USDA diet pyramid promotes the idea of categorizing all fats as equal, and their intake should be limited.

Although the USDA diet pyramid model was considered a very healthy approach to adopt from its inception till 2005, however, the Mediterranean diet pyramid has grown substantial support globally and gained the trust of millions of people and experts across the world. The main factor for this success can be classified as the ability to mould the Mediterranean diet pyramid into various tastes and dietary choices due to its highly flexible, systematic buildup. The preferences with the Mediterranean diet pyramid can range from gluten-free, vegan free, and much more. Irrespective of the fact that the Mediterranean diet pyramid was punished in the 90s, the diet pyramid still represents and describes present-day beliefs and practices that comprise together to form the Mediterranean diet. The Mediterranean diet pyramid allows focusing on formulating healthy eating patterns by including nutrition-rich, dense foods instead of focusing on what is not allowed and what cannot be eaten.

The Health Benefits of the Mediterranean Diet

The Mediterranean diet is famous for its highly advantageous and life-saving health benefits. The prime reason for the popularity of the Mediterranean diet is the numerous health benefits that make it stand apart from the rest of its competitors. Some of the vital health benefits of the diet are as follows:

1. Memory Preservation

The Mediterranean diet is very effective in the memory preservation and reducing the risk of cognitive declines. The major reason for this is considered that the diet is affluent in its fat content. This fat content is very beneficial for the human brain and also reduces the risk of dementia. A scientific study stated that the Mediterranean diet plan would significantly lower the risk of cognitive decline by 40%.

2. Reduced Cardiovascular Diseases

The Mediterranean diet is very effective in lowering cardiac-related risk factors like cholesterol, triglycerides, and high BP. This is the prime factor for having a reduced risk of cardiovascular diseases like coronary heart diseases, myocardial infarction or heart attack, and strokes.

3. Strong Bones

The Mediterranean diet an abundance of olive oil in its food list. Olive oil is known to increase the maturity and proliferation of the bone cells that results in effective bone preservation, and strengthens bone density. Moreover, the diet habits of the Mediterranean diet plan are known to lower the risk of osteoporosis.

4. Blood Sugar Control

The Mediterranean diet is very effective in controlling diabetes and blood sugar. A study also showed that it could be effective in reversing type 2 diabetes. Furthermore, it can improve blood sugar control and cardiac issues in people already suffering from them. The diet followers showed a lesser urge to get medical treatment, effective weight loss, and improved blood sugar control in comparison to low-fat diet followers.

5. Cancer Prevention

The Mediterranean diet is known to lower the risk of terminal cancer by 13%. The diet is effective in lowering the chances of cancers like breast cancer, colorectal cancer, head cancer, liver cancer, gastric cancer, neck cancer, prostate cancer.

6. Anti-Depression Effect

The diet is also known for having anti-depressant properties. A study in 2013 showed that diet followers had approximately 99% lower risk of getting into depression than other people.

How to Get Started with the Mediterranean Diet

The entire idea of the Mediterranean diet is to adopt the model diet that is prevalent in the Mediterranean region. The Mediterranean diet pyramid acts as the basis to formulate the list of Dos and Don'ts when it comes to starting your diet in an effective manner. However, for your easiness, there is a golden to remember, i.e., Fill half your plate with fruits and veggies, one-quarter of your plate with healthy proteins, and one-quarter of your plate with whole grains. However, for a better understanding and effective implementation of the Mediterranean diet, follow the following section profoundly to have promising results in less time.

1. Focus Whole Foods

It should be understood that processed foods are not included in the Mediterranean diet. If your food is packaged, check the list thoroughly. Prefer opting for foods having 2 to 3 whole food ingredients like oats or bulgur. Whole foods can be veggies, whole grains, fish, fruits, nuts, olive oil, and legumes.

2. Veggies Are the Prime Ingredient

The main focus of your diet should be veggies and fruits, i.e., 7 to 10 servings of both veggies and fruits on a daily basis. If you take 3 to 5 servings of veggies and fruits, that too will help you in cardiovascular complications. However, the more, the better. Manage to add veggies in your recipes by innovative ways like loading your sandwich with cucumber and avocado, choosing apple with nut butter instead of crackers, and combining spinach with eggs.

3. Fish as an Alternative for Red Meat

The Mediterranean diet includes fatty fish like tuna, herring, salmon, and mackerel, which are excellent sources of protein and omega-3 fatty acids. Omega-3 fatty acids are known to improve good cholesterol levels and reduce inflammation in the body. Shellfish and whitefish are also considered effective protein sources. However, they do lack in the omega-3 fatty content. Processed and red meats are eaten very rarely, on special occasions. You can opt for eggs, cheese, turkey, yogurt, and chicken in moderate quantities on weekends or even daily.

4. Start Using Olive Oil

The prime fat source in the Mediterranean diet is olive oil. Net fat is not as crucial as the overall type of fat. The Mediterranean diet focuses on consuming mono-unsaturated and poly-unsaturated fats that are good for health. It also minimizes the usage of trans fats and saturated fats. The latter is known to increased LDL or harmful cholesterol levels. You can switch to olive oil instead of butter for a healthy lifestyle with the Mediterranean diet.

5. Reconsider Your Diary Intake

You should opt for a flavorful cheese in a very limited or moderate quantity. Go for strong-flavored cheeses like Parmesan or feta instead of processed cheeses. You can go for Greek, plain, and fermented yogurt and

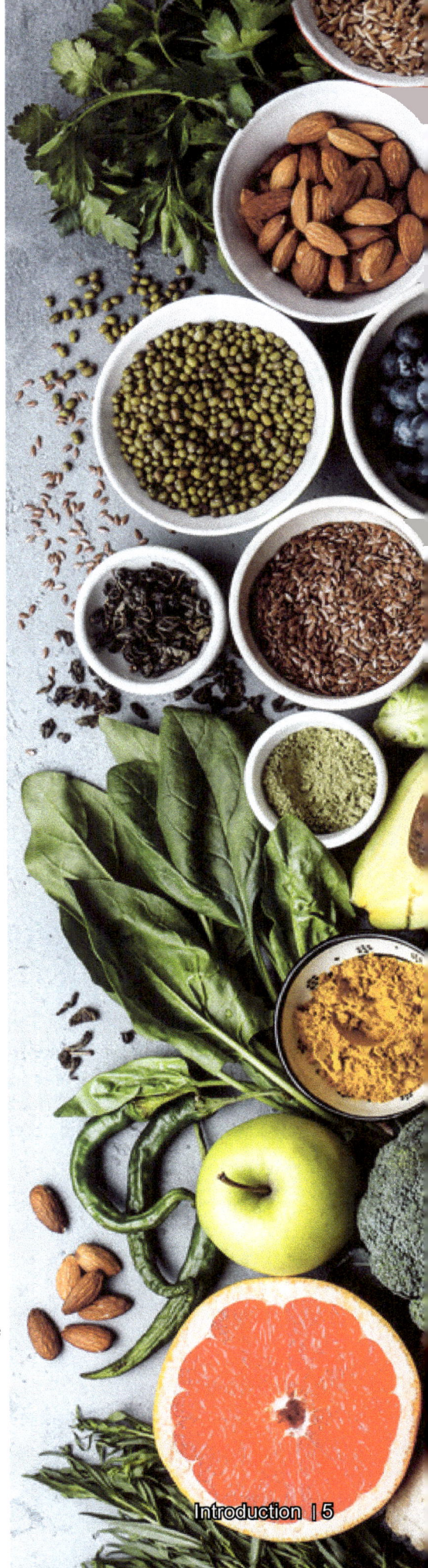

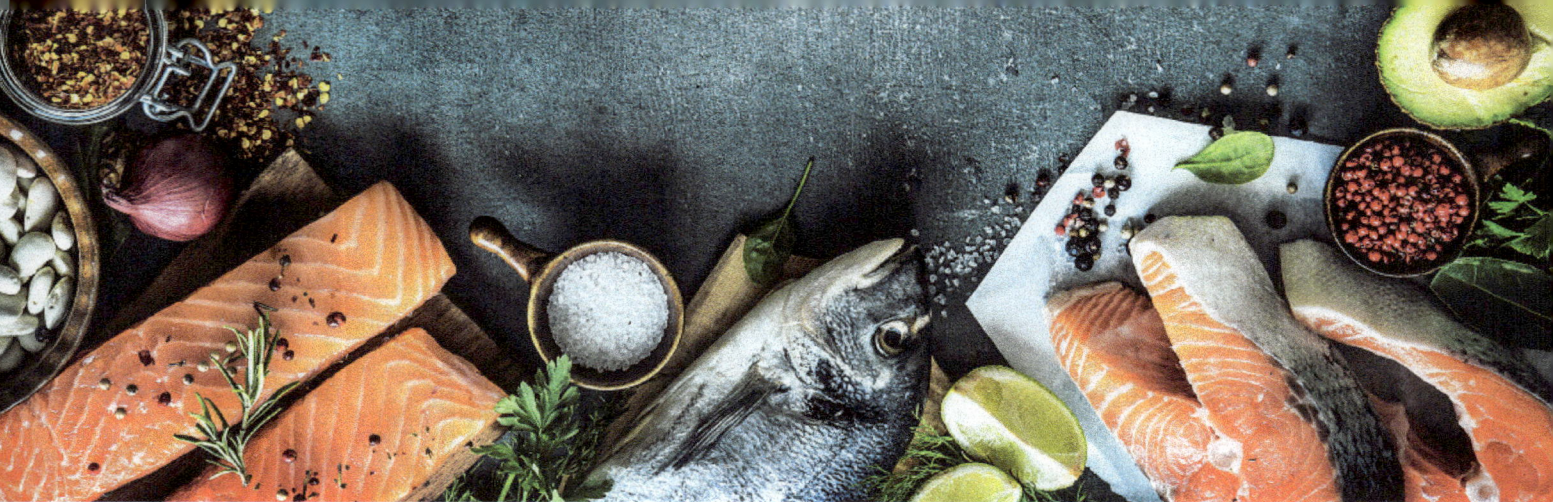

avoid any high-sugar yogurts, as high sugar is a big no for good health.

6. Substitute Refined Grains with Whole Grains

Substitute pasta and rice for whole grains like farro, barley, and bulgur. There are a lot of benefits of whole grains, and they are a significant portion of the Mediterranean diet. They lower cholesterol levels, have high vitamin B and fibre, and improve blood sugar and overall weight loss. You can also go for legumes and beans.

7. Nuts as Snacks

Nuts are having high quantities of poly and mono-unsaturated fats like avocados and olive oil. They also offer fibre and protein, therefore, offering the perfect nutrient-trio for stabilizing blood sugar, reduction in inflammation, remaining full, and lower down bad cholesterol. You can have a ¼ cup of nuts as a snack between lunch and dinner. You can go pairing them with veggies and fruits to remain full for long. Walnuts are a great source of omega-3 fatty acids, so it is also a great choice.

8. Avoid Sugar Mostly

Crackers, sugars, processed cookies, and refined flours are certainly not a part of the Mediterranean diet. You can opt for ice cream and cookies on special or rare occasions. The Mediterranean culture has baklava and gelato as sweet in moderate quantity. Usually, figs and dates are used for killing sugar cravings in the Mediterranean region.

9. Moderate Red Wine

If you drink, 10 ounces of red wine per day is allowed for men. Whereas for women, the allowed quantity is 5 ounces. However, if you are not into drinking, don't start it with the diet as it is not recommended.

Mediterranean Diet Food List to Follow

Foods to Eat

The allowed food list for the Mediterranean Diet is given below category wise. However, it is essential to consider the following simple approach while considering the Mediterranean diet:
1. Eat moderate poultry and dairy products.
2. Eat red meat on special occasions.
3. Eat veggies, fruits, nuts, seeds, legumes, and other products in abundance.

Fruits & Veggies

- Oranges
- Apricots
- Peaches
- Grapes
- Yams
- Greens like kale, arugula, collards, and spinach
- Cabbage
- Onions
- Berries
- Pears
- Dates
- Cherries
- Potatoes
- Peppers
- Beets
- Bananas
- Avocado
- Figs
- Turnips
- Tomatoes
- Brussels sprouts
- Apples
- Clementines
- Melons
- Artichokes
- Peas
- Zucchini

Whole Grains

You can match and mix them for an easy side dish, simple stir-fries, or even grain-bowl bases.
- Rye
- Pasta
- Couscous
- Brown rice
- Bulgur
- Buckwheat
- Corn
- Oats
- Barley
- Whole-grain bread
- Farro

Fish & Seafood

Fish & seafood are a prime part of the Mediterranean diet. You should consume more of it instead of other meat sources.
- Herring
- Mussels
- Salmon
- Sardines
- Clams
- Mackerel
- Trout
- Shrimps
- Other seafood of your choice
- Crabs
- Tuna

Poultry

You should eat these lean meats & other poultry items in a moderate amount.
- Turkey
- Chicken eggs
- Chicken
- Turkey eggs
- Duck
- Quail eggs

Meats

You can consume the following protein-rich meats intermittently. You can make a combo of whole grains, veggies, and a small portion of meats for a great Mediterranean diet.
- Beef
- Pork
- Lamb, only a few times every month or even less

Dairy Products

We recommend you using grass-fed and pasture-raised dairy in a moderate amount.
- Greek yogurt
- Plain yogurt
- Unprocessed cheese options like brie, Parmesan, feta, and ricotta

Legumes, Seeds, and Nuts

You can have them as snacks, salad toppings, and much more in your desired recipes.
- Macadamia nuts
- Hazelnuts
- Chickpeas
- Sesame seeds
- Pine nuts
- Sunflower seeds
- Almonds
- Cashews
- Pumpkin seeds
- Fava

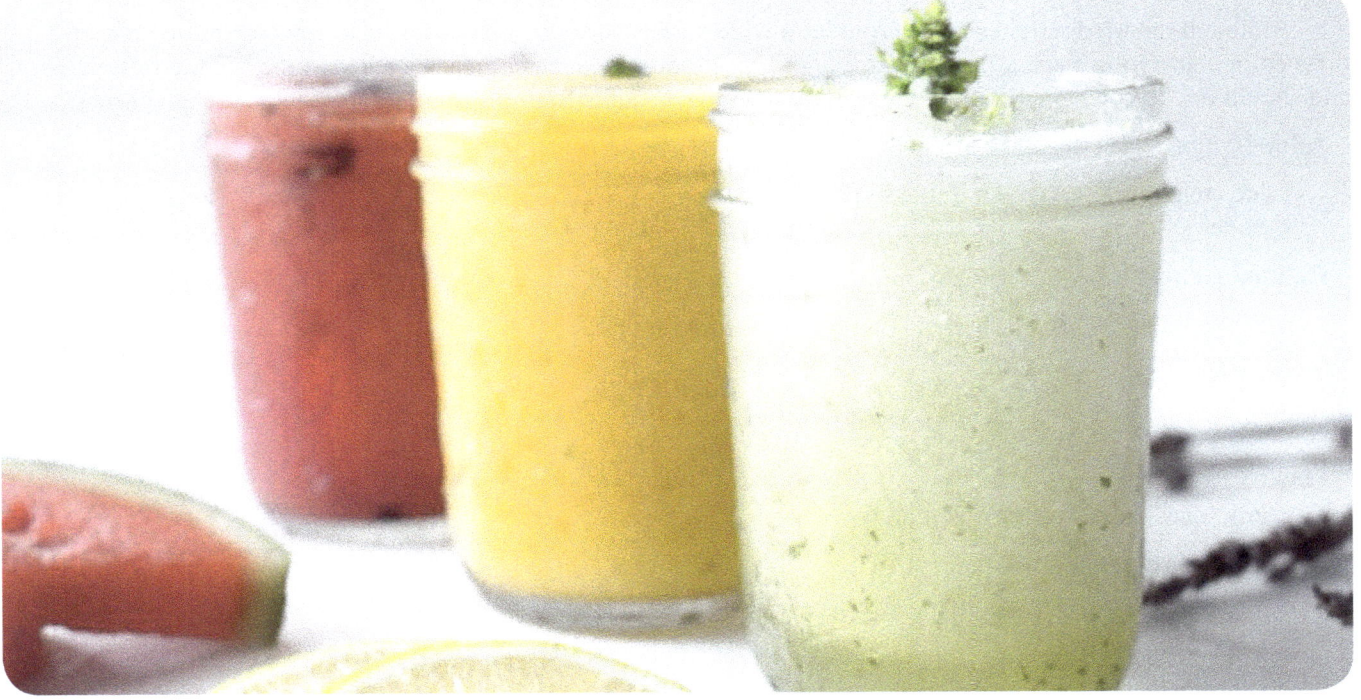

Introduction | 7

Spices & Herbs

You can add more to your spices and herbs than salt. You can have both fresh and dry herbs on the Mediterranean diet.

- Nutmeg
- Parsley
- Mint
- Pepper
- Basil
- Rosemary
- Cinnamon
- Garlic
- Sage
- Oregano
- Tarragon

Oils

Always prefer mono-unsaturated and poly-unsaturated oils.
- Olive oil
- Soybean oil
- Canola oil
- Flaxseed oil
- Avocado oil

Beverages & Drinks

- Red wine in the mentioned quantities (Only if you drink)
- Water
- Tea and coffee (no or very minimal sugar)

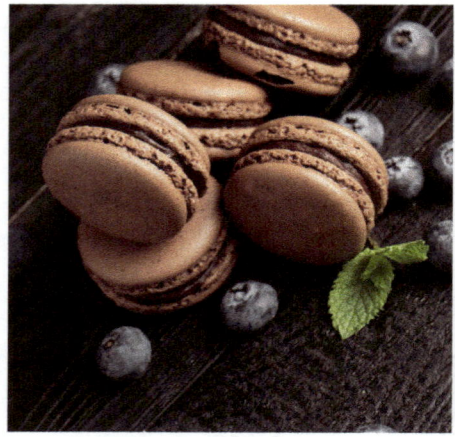 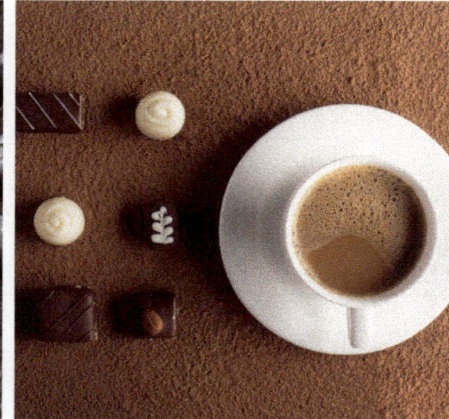 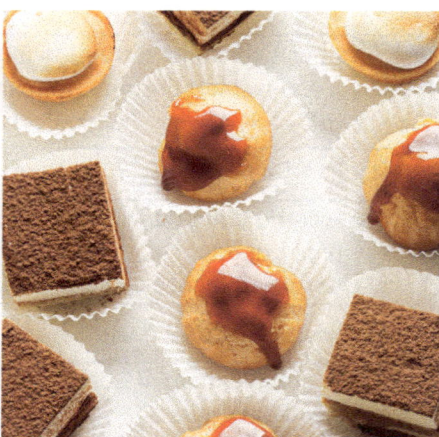

Foods to Avoid

Although the Mediterranean diet provides a wide variety of food choices for its followers, it also restricts them from consuming a specific group of foods. These foods are against the very ethos of the Mediterranean diet and should not be consumed at all to experience the most benefits from the diet. Some of them are as follows:

Added Sugars

- Ice cream
- Soda
- Table sugar
- Other similar items
- Candies
- Pastries

Refined Grains

- White bread
- Pasta (containing refined wheat)

Trans Fats

- Margarine
- Processed fats

Processed Meats

- Processed sausages
- Hot dogs

Refined & Saturated Oils

- Palm Oil
- Palm Kernel Oil
- Hydrogenated Oils

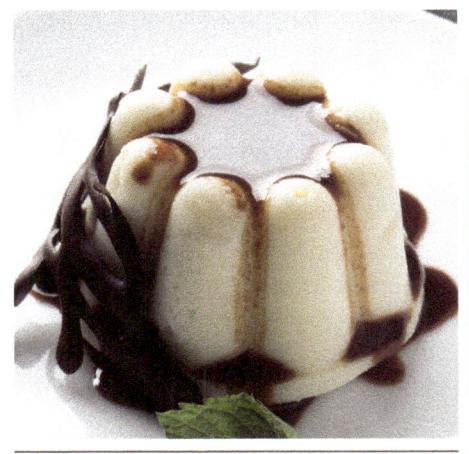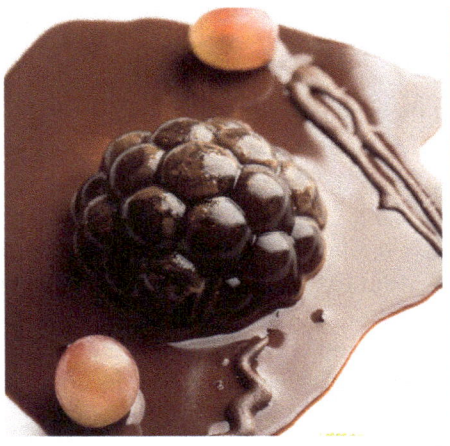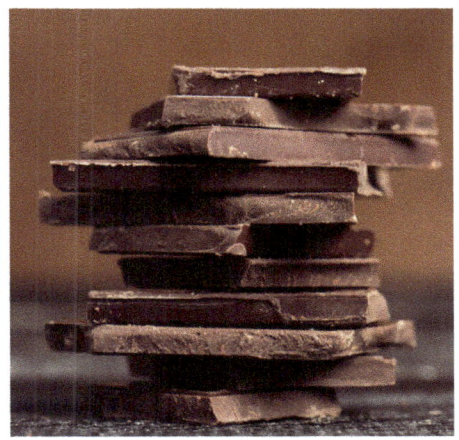

Highly Processed Foods
- Tinned veggies
- Biscuits and other similar products

Beverages & Drinks
- High-sugar drinks
- Fruit juices with added sugar
- Sugar-sweetened beverages

Shopping Guide for the Mediterranean Diet

The following guidelines can be beneficial when you are going shopping out for your Mediterranean diet. These guidelines can be a game-changer in the long run for a successful Mediterranean diet. They are as follows:

1. Fish Counter
It is imperative to include healthy fats in your diet. You can quickly go for farmed algae-fed salmon. They are known to have higher omega-3 fatty acids than wild fish. It will provide you with ample nutrition like wild fish.

2. Getting Fresh Herbs
Herbs are the best flavoring ingredients without having a fear of increased calories. You should always opt for the freshest herbs available in the supermarket to make your diet more nutritious and add more flavor to your favorite recipes. Cilantro and basil are great fresh seasonal herbs that are relatively inexpensive.

3. Go for Honey
Honey is the best option to add some sugar to your recipes. So when you are going out shopping, never forget to get a stock of honey to add some sweetness to your life. Honey itself is having a lot of medical benefits, and its combo with the Mediterranean diet is going to be amazing.

4. Variety of Grain
Grains are primarily considered an essential part of the Mediterranean diet. It would be regarded as best if you went for unprocessed whole grains when doing groceries in the supermarket. Always check the packaging for the origin of the ingredients to verify if they are unprocessed or not. You can go through the nutrition table to see if they are whole grains or not like whole-wheat, oats, rye-berries, etc.

5. Prefer Opting for Produce
As explained earlier, veggies and fruits constitute most of the Mediterranean diet. It can be easily understood that when you shop groceries, most of what you will be buying will be produce. It would be

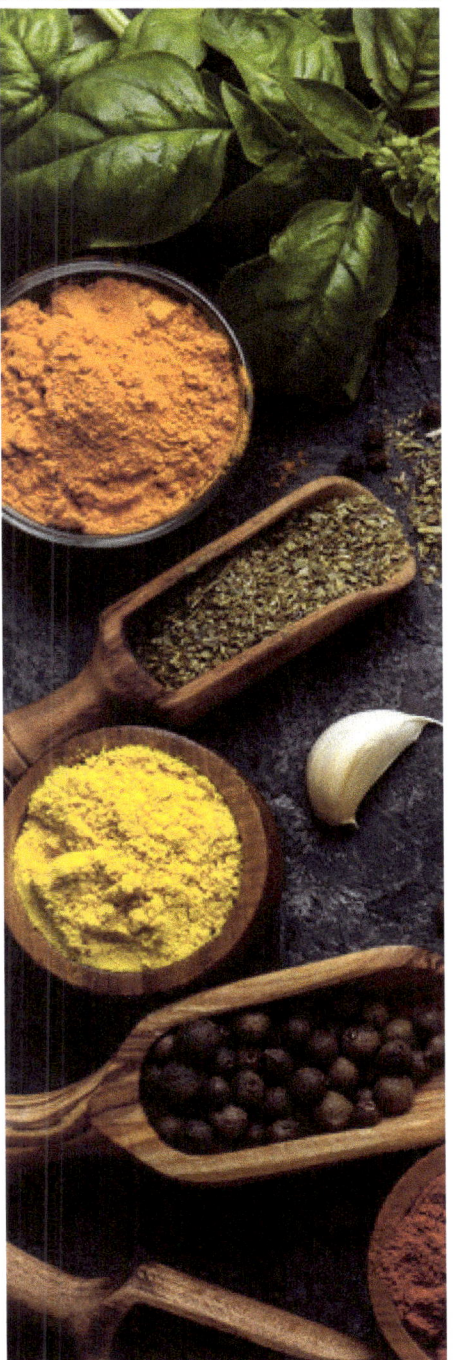

best if you always went for seasoned and locally grown veggies and fruits as they will be having a higher chance of being fresher, and they will probably cost lesser.

6. The Frozen Section
Generally, fresh foods are frozen at their peak freshness, which is why frozen food are likely as nutritious as frozen ones. You can go for frozen foods for breakfast like cereals and yogurt. You can also grab some frozen fish fillets, or frozen veggies with sauces.

7. Going for the Right Seeds & Nuts
Mostly the varieties of nuts and seeds available in supermarkets are salted, sugar-coated, or covered in chocolate. It would be best if you always went for plain seeds and nuts that can be either roasted or raw.

8. The Dairy Section
You can go for Greek yogurt, or unprocessed cheese choices like ricotta and feta, etc. Dairy products are consumed in moderate amounts and you can choose between both low-fat and high-fat choices. High-fat dairy will have more calories but you can feel fuller with them.

9. Buying the Right Oil
Although the most famously used oil on the Mediterranean diet is extra-virgin olive oil | however, the oil is very unstable at high temperatures, so it is best for drizzling over prepared recipes or salad dressing. You can also opt for using regular olive oil or even canola oil if you are going for high-heat recipes.

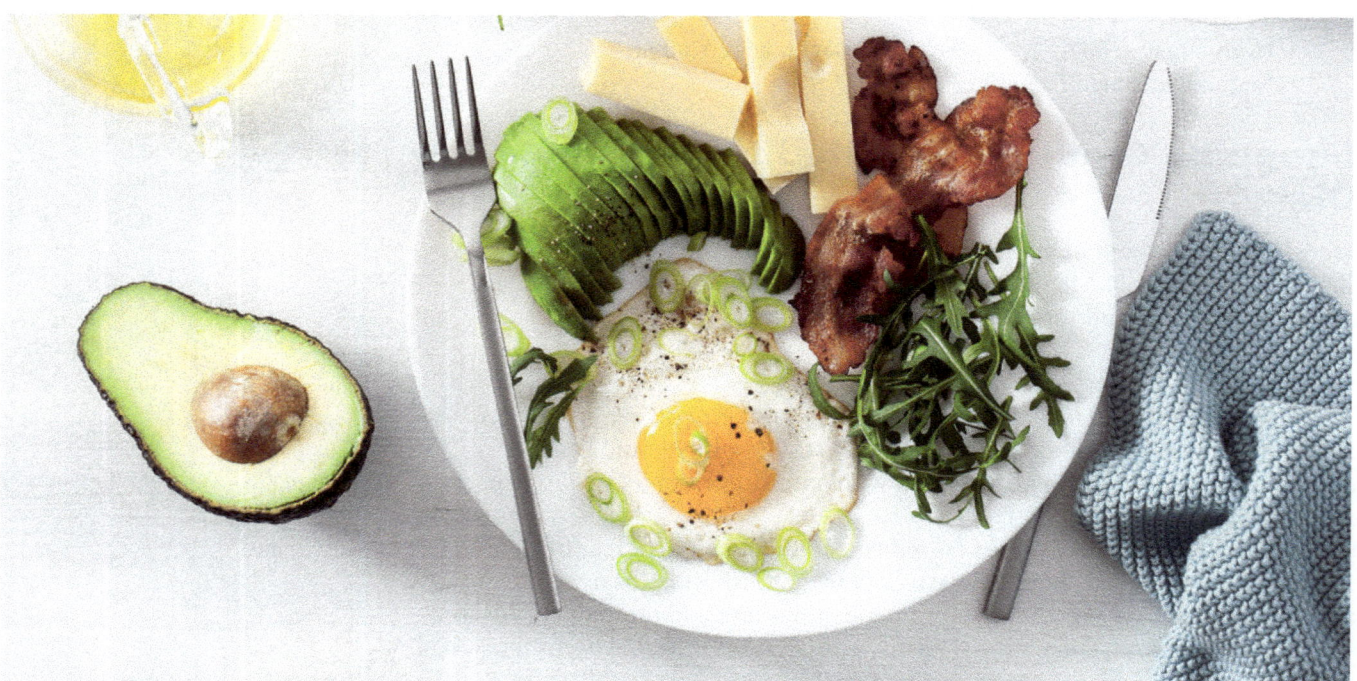

Tips for Success

For an effective and more successful Mediterranean diet, the following tips and tricks should be followed:

1. Increasing Veggie Intake
It is generally understood that increased veggies mean a healthier lifestyle. Various studies verify that plant-heavy diets are more beneficial than other diets. Different studies ponder that having 7 or more servings of veggies and fruits daily can significantly lower the risk of heart issues.

2. Have More Legumes
The most protein-rich ingredient in the Mediterranean diet is legumes. Furthermore, they are also excellent sources of dietary fibre. One cup of navy beans will provide you more dietary fibre than more protein than two eggs and seven slices of whole-wheat bread. So eat more legumes.

3. Enough Intake of Fish & Seafood
Vitamin B & D, selenium, and proteins are highly available in seafood and fish. A study explains that a 2 pounds of fish intake can lower the risk of death by 12%. Fatty fishes are a must on the Mediterranean diet.

4. Usage of Olive Oil
The most subtle way of a successful Mediterranean diet is to replace all oils, butter, and margarine with olive

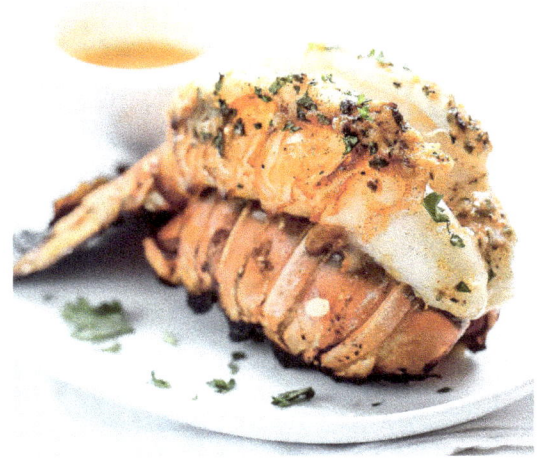

oil. Olive oil contains HDL cholesterol producing mono-saturated fats. HDL cholesterol is known as good cholesterol and is known to prevent heart strokes.

5. Fruits as Desserts

Fruits are having high fibre content, low fat, and effective antioxidants. Fruit consumption is known to reduce diabetes risk. Moreover, apples and pears are known to lower the risk of heart diseases. You can use fruits as snacks or even desserts in the Mediterranean diet.

6. Diary as a Garnish

Dairy products that are allowed in the Mediterranean diet can be used in small amounts for garnishing. Dairy products can lower the risk of diabetes, metabolic syndrome, obesity, heart complications, and diabetes.

7. Reduce Meat Intake

The Mediterranean diet is not focused on having meat in larger quantity apart from special occasions and events. The meat used in the Mediterranean diet is pasture-raised, grass-fed, having increased CLA and omega-3 fatty acids.

8. Increase Seasonings

Unlike the American diet, the Mediterranean diet is focused on herbs and seasonings instead of salt. Consider garlic | it can lower harmful cholesterol levels, increase immunity, reduce the risk of cancer. Herbs are known as antioxidants and can reduce the risk of various serious diseases.

9. Socialize

The concept of fast food is out of the question in the Mediterranean diet. Instead, you should dine together with your friends and family to make your eating habits more social.

10. Go for Meal Planning

Meal planning can prove your Mediterranean diet to be very successful as you can avoid last minute rush to the stores to grab missing ingredients. You can also avoid eating restricted food if you plan out your meals thoroughly. The coming section will discuss meal planning in detail.

Mediterranean Meal Planning

There are numerous benefits of meal planning while following the Mediterranean diet. These benefits can help you in adopting the diet befittingly and provide you with maximum support to achieve success on the Mediterranean diet. They are as follows:

1. Time-Saving

Meal planning on the weekends can prove to be very time-saving and helps you in managing your time effectively. A considerable amount of time goes into what to eat, going for groceries, cooking your food, and then doing cleanups. Meal planning can help you save any last-minute trips to the supermarket and keep your meals more organized. It also allows you a lot in overspending and wandering in the supermarket.

2. Effective Portion Control

If you are following the Mediterranean diet for

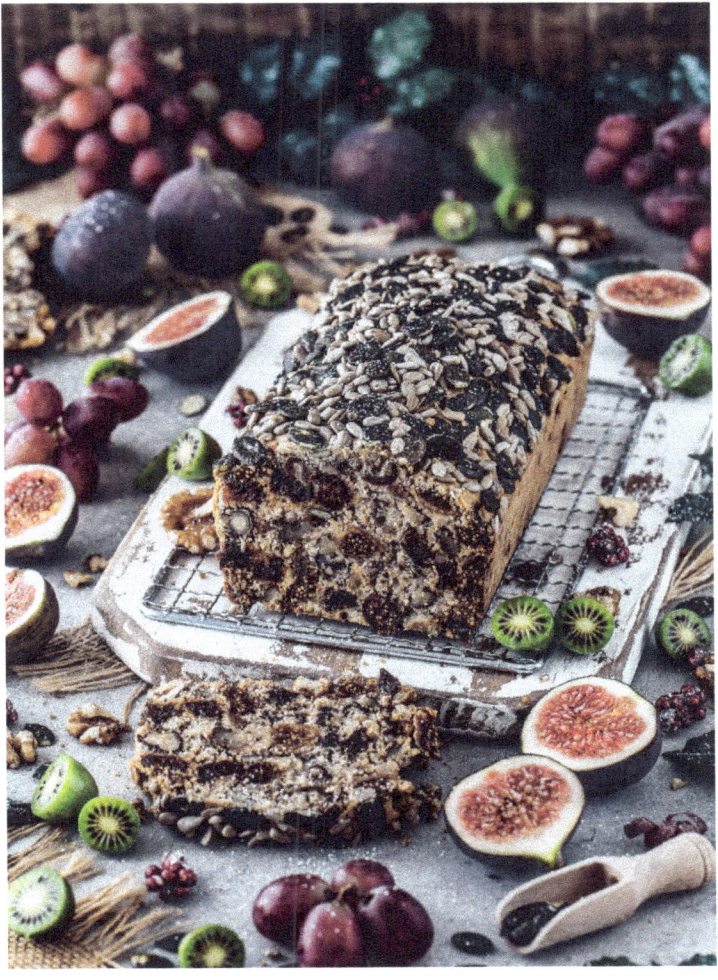

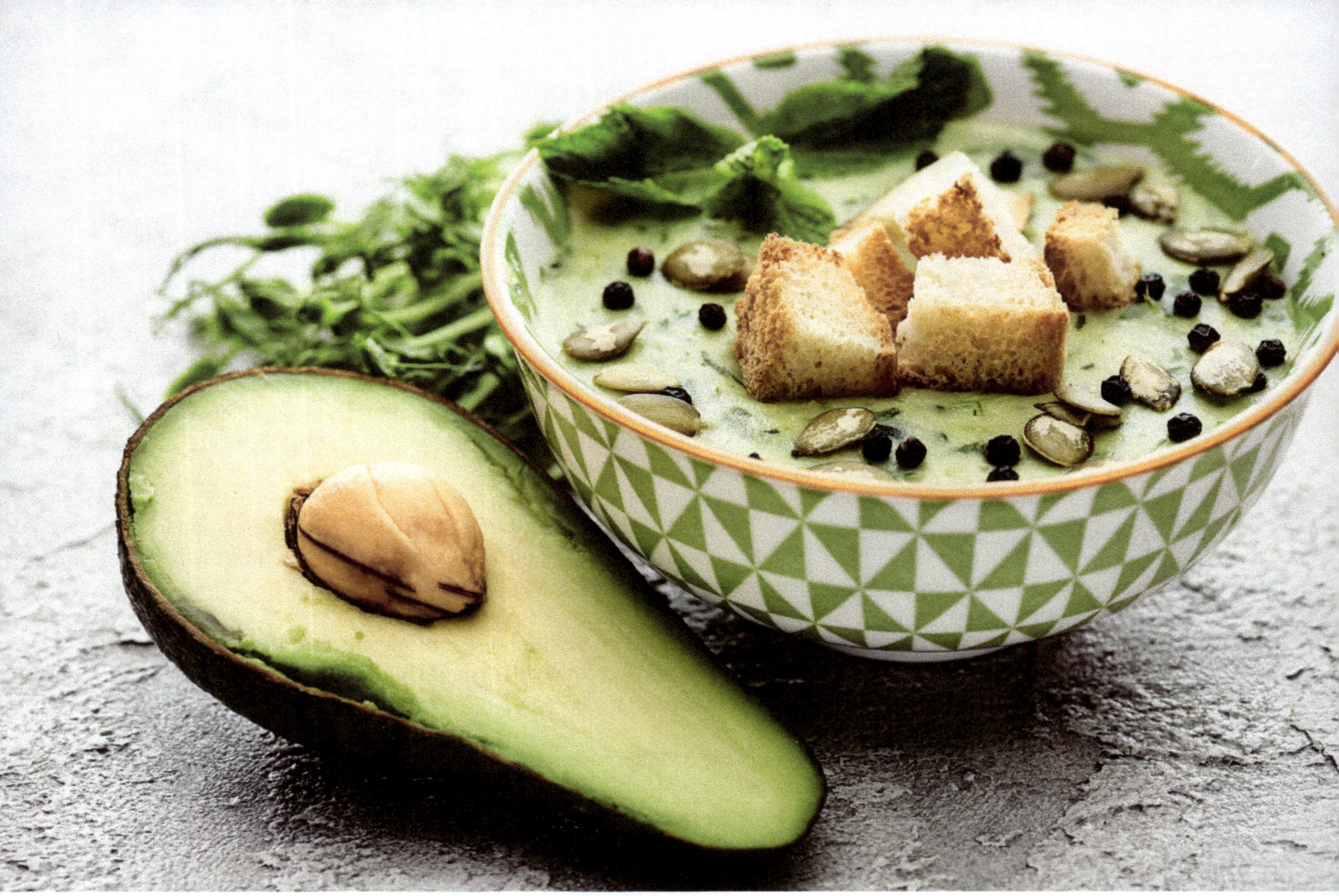

weight-loss plans, meal prepping is an effective approach along with meal planning. It can help you control your food portions and stop you from overeating.

3. Reduction in Food Wastage

Meal planning can be very helpful in thoroughly cutting down the amount of food going into waste. We all are somewhat guilty of food waste at some point in our lives. Thoroughly planning what ingredients you require and how much your portion sizes will be can be very effective in considerably lowering down the amount of food going into waste.

4. Stress Relieving

If you opt for meal planning, you will undoubtedly avoid the stress of last-minute cooking and instead have your meals organized beforehand. Planning your dinner after coming from work can become a significant burden and cause a lot of stress. If you go for meal planning on the Mediterranean diet, you can pre-organize your meals and don't burden yourself with the stress of cooking in the last hours when you are all tired from work.

5. Economical

Saving money is the most appealing part of any plan. Meal planning can save you a lot of money by making you aware of the ingredients you need for the recipes you have planned. It will avoid you overbuying things which you don't need at the supermarket. You can also slash down the money you spend on dine outs and takeaways on the Mediterranean diet with meal planning. It will also make you financially aware of the overall cost of your diet and how it can be optimized more effectively.

6. Avoiding Unhealthy Items

Meal planning can easily make your meal options healthier after thoroughly sorting out the right and most healthy nutrients for your recipes. Having an already planned meal at home will let you avoid the cravings of dining outs and takeaways and enable you to eat healthier and nutritious homemade food. Stress and tiredness can become significant factors in opting for easy unhealthy food choices, which are hazardous for your Mediterranean diet.

7. Having More Variety

Meal planning can be very beneficial in figuring out a thorough variety of different recipes for all your meals. Moreover, you can also avoid making similar recipes over and over again. Meal planning can also enable you to do new experiments with your ingredients and prepare jaw licking recipe for yourself and your loved ones.

Frequently Asked Questions (FAQs)

1. Is Mediterranean Diet just any other fad diet?

No, it is not the case. In fact, the Mediterranean diet is not just merely a plan | it is a complete lifestyle. It cannot be classified as a temporary diet approach towards losing weight. Instead, it is a lifelong habitual healthy approach to life. This way of eating is known to be sustainable and is having comprehensive health benefits.

2. Is workout effective with the Mediterranean Diet?

Well, the Mediterranean diet is not about eating seeds and nuts, having red wine, and taking a rest. Physical activities and workout is an essential part of the Mediterranean diet. In fact, the Mediterranean diet pyramid also includes exercise as a necessary aspect of the diet. You have to perform exercise and physical activities along with the Mediterranean diet to achieve the most success with the diet.

3. What about the calorie intake?

The Mediterranean diet lets you eat slower and enjoy your food. It makes you feel full sooner, and this happens with the passage of time. Despite this, you have to be careful about your food portion and sizes to avoid overeating. You can do a thorough meal planning which can curb your cravings and overeating. You can also consult your dietitian to provide you with more effective information on your calorie intake on the basis of your physical features and your body requirements.

21 Days Mediterranean diet Meal Plan

DAYS	BREAKFAST	LUNCH	DINNER	SNACK/DESSERT	REMINDER
1	Spinach Pie	Mediterranean Quinoa and Garbanzo Salad	Chicken with Olives and Capers	Mediterranean Trail Mix	Moderate Exercise; A Glass of Wine.
2	Fig and Ricotta Toast with Walnuts and Honey	Sautéed Mushroom, Onion, and Pecorino Romano Panini	Shrimp Pasta with Basil and Mushrooms	Air Fryer Popcorn with Garlic Salt	Moderate Exercise; A Glass of Wine.
3	Blueberry-Banana Bowl with Quinoa	Sweet Veggie-Stuffed Peppers	Spiced Oven-Baked Meatballs with Tomato Sauce	Poached Pears with Greek Yogurt and Pistachio	Moderate Exercise; A Glass of Wine.
4	Greek Egg and Tomato Scramble	Classic Margherita Pizza	Mediterranean Garlic and Herb-Roasted Cod	Fruit Compote	Moderate Exercise; A Glass of Wine.
5	Greek Yogurt Parfait with Granola	Moroccan-Style Couscous	Mediterranean Roasted Turkey Breast	Burrata Caprese Stack	Moderate Exercise; A Glass of Wine.

DAYS	BREAKFAST	LUNCH	DINNER	SNACK/ DESSERT	REMINDER
6	Garlicky Beans and Greens with Polenta	Superfood Salmon Salad Bowl	Moroccan-Spiced Chicken Thighs with Saffron Basmati Rice	Crispy Spiced Chickpeas	Moderate Exercise; A Glass of Wine.
7	Egg and Pepper Pita	Moroccan Date Pilaf	Shrimp Paella	Greek Yogurt with Honey and Pomegranates	Moderate Exercise; A Glass of Wine.
8	Strawberry Collagen Smoothie	Tuscan Kale Salad with Anchovies	Pork Casserole with Fennel and Potatoes	Figs with Mascarpone and Honey	Moderate Exercise; A Glass of Wine.
9	Spinach and Feta Frittata	Grilled Eggplant Rolls	Bomba Chicken with Chickpeas	Cheese-Stuffed Dates	Moderate Exercise; A Glass of Wine.
10	Whole Wheat Banana-Walnut Bread	Bomba Chicken with Chickpeas	Mediterranean Garlic and Herb-Roasted Cod	Baked Italian Spinach and Ricotta Balls	Moderate Exercise; A Glass of Wine.
11	Buckwheat Porridge with Fresh Fruit	Roasted Vegetable Bocadillo with Romesco Sauce	Chicken with Olives and Capers	Toasted Almonds with Honey	Moderate Exercise; A Glass of Wine.
12	Greek Yogurt Parfait with Granola	Turkey and Provolone Panini with Roasted Peppers and Onions	Cheesy Spinach Pies	Pears Poached in Pomegranate and Wine	Moderate Exercise; A Glass of Wine.
13	Spinach Pie	Shrimp and Asparagus Risotto	Baked Red Snapper with Potatoes and Tomatoes	Crispy Spiced Chickpeas	Moderate Exercise; A Glass of Wine.
14	Savory Cottage Cheese Breakfast Bowl	Mediterranean Pasta Salad	Chicken Avgolemono	Mediterranean Trail Mix	Moderate Exercise; A Glass of Wine.
15	Spanish Tortilla with Potatoes and Peppers	Tunisian Bean Soup with Poached Eggs	Mediterranean Garlic and Herb-Roasted Cod	Light and Lemony Olive Oil Cupcakes	Moderate Exercise; A Glass of Wine.
16	Egg in a "Pepper Hole" with Avocado	Meatballs in Creamy Almond Sauce	Kale, Chickpea, and Chicken Stew	Baked Italian Spinach and Ricotta Balls	Moderate Exercise; A Glass of Wine.

DAYS	BREAKFAST	LUNCH	DINNER	SNACK/ DESSERT	REMINDER
17	Strawberry Collagen Smoothie	Walnut and Freekeh Pilaf	Poached Octopus	Cheese-Stuffed Dates	Moderate Exercise; A Glass of Wine.
18	Mediterranean Breakfast Pita Sandwiches	Salmon with Tarragon-Dijon Sauce	Mediterranean Roasted Turkey Breast	Crunchy Sesame Cookies	Moderate Exercise; A Glass of Wine.
19	Blueberry-Banana Bowl with Quinoa	Taverna-Style Greek Salad	Hearty Stewed Beef in Tomato Sauce	Fruit Compote	Moderate Exercise; A Glass of Wine.
20	Egg Salad with Red Pepper and Dill	Cheesy Spinach Pies	Mediterranean Garlic and Herb-Roasted Cod	Air Fryer Popcorn with Garlic Salt	Moderate Exercise; A Glass of Wine.
21	Garlicky Beans and Greens with Polenta	Chicken Cutlets with Greek Salsa	Shrimp Paella	Mediterranean Trail Mix	Moderate Exercise; A Glass of Wine.

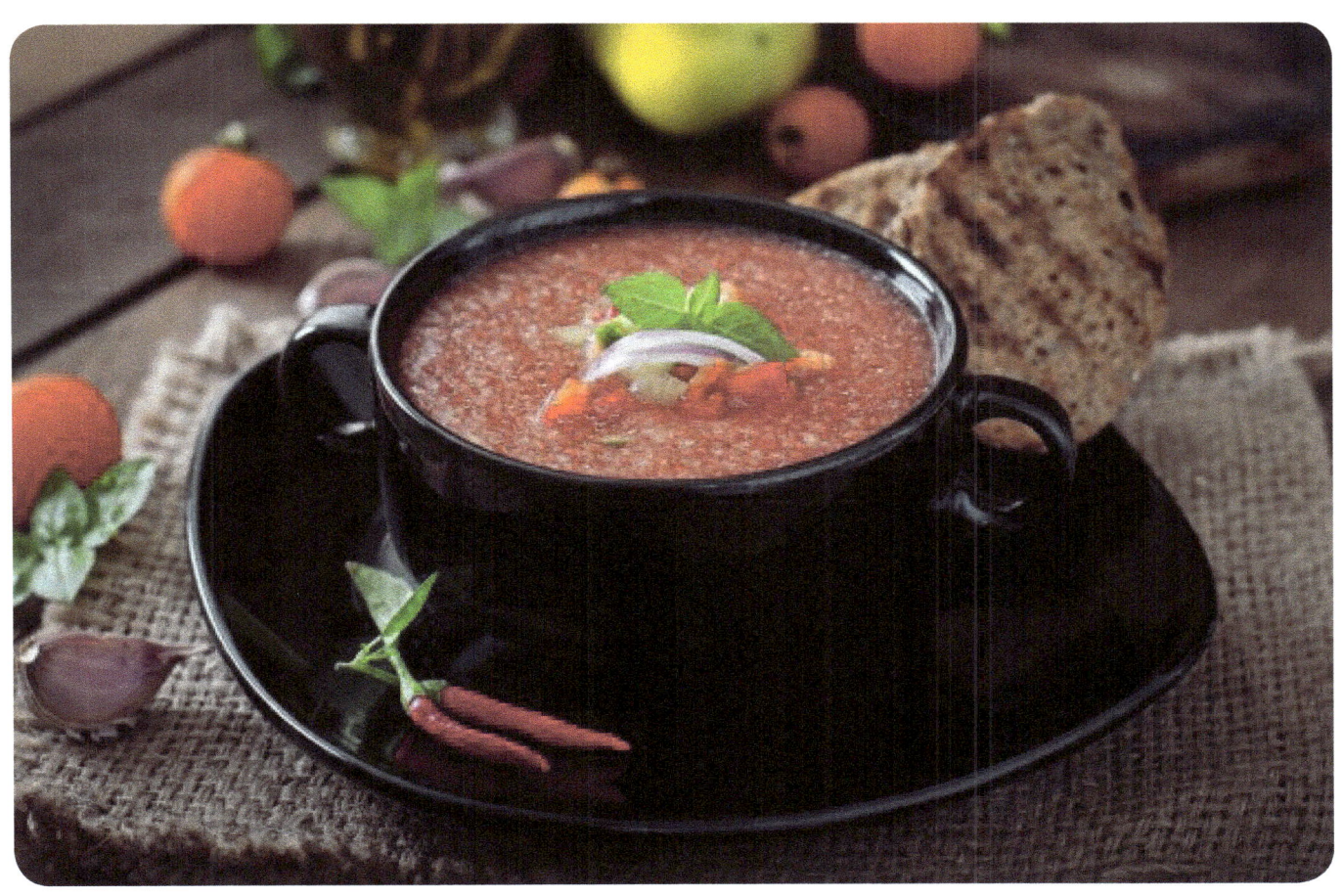

Chapter 1   Basics

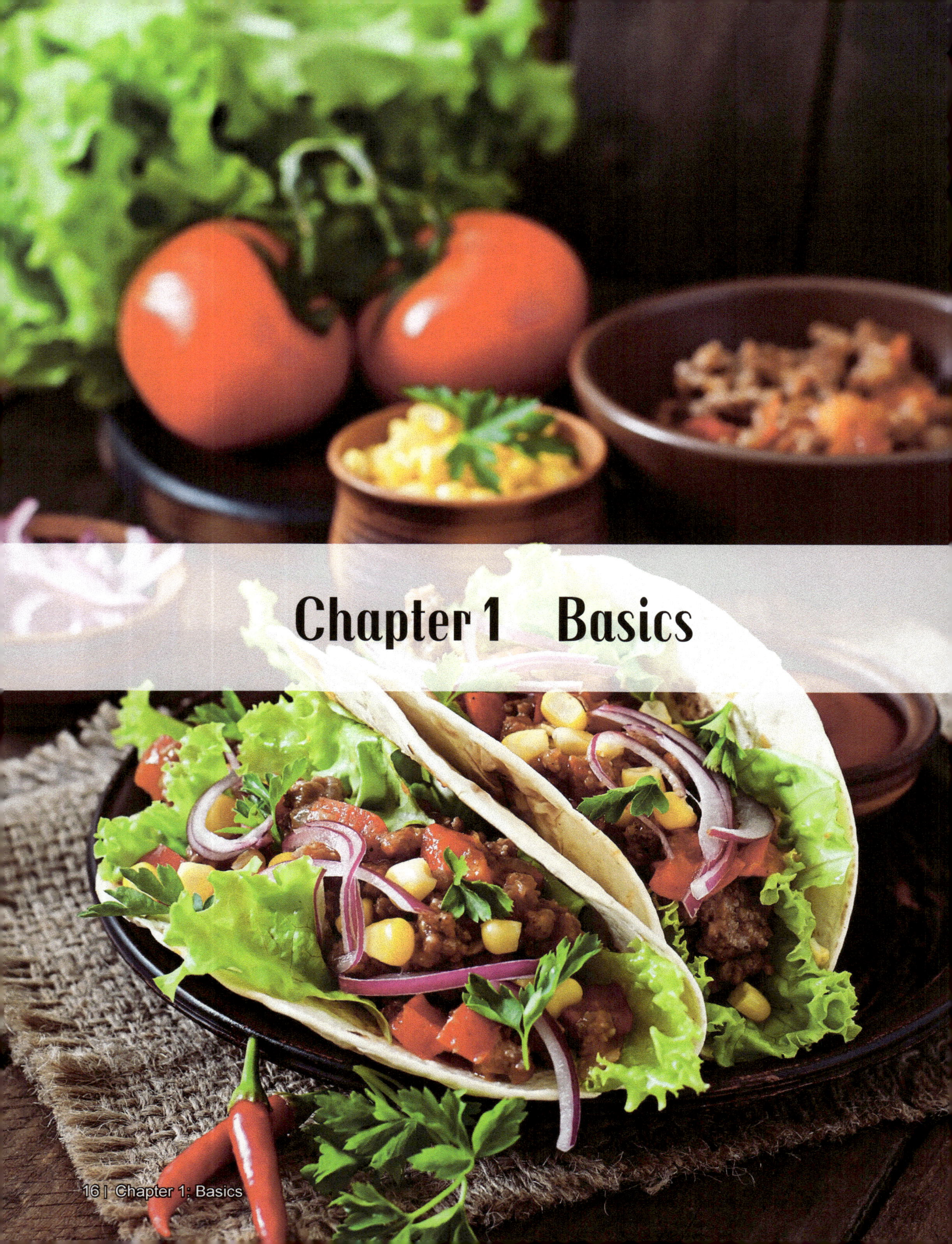

1. **Baked Fish with Olives** 18
2. **Pan-Seared Shrimp Skewers** 18
3. **Shrimp Saganaki** 18
4. **Cod and Potatoes in Avgolemono** 19
5. **Tomato and White Beans with Garlic Shrimp** 19
6. **Foil-Baked Fish** 19

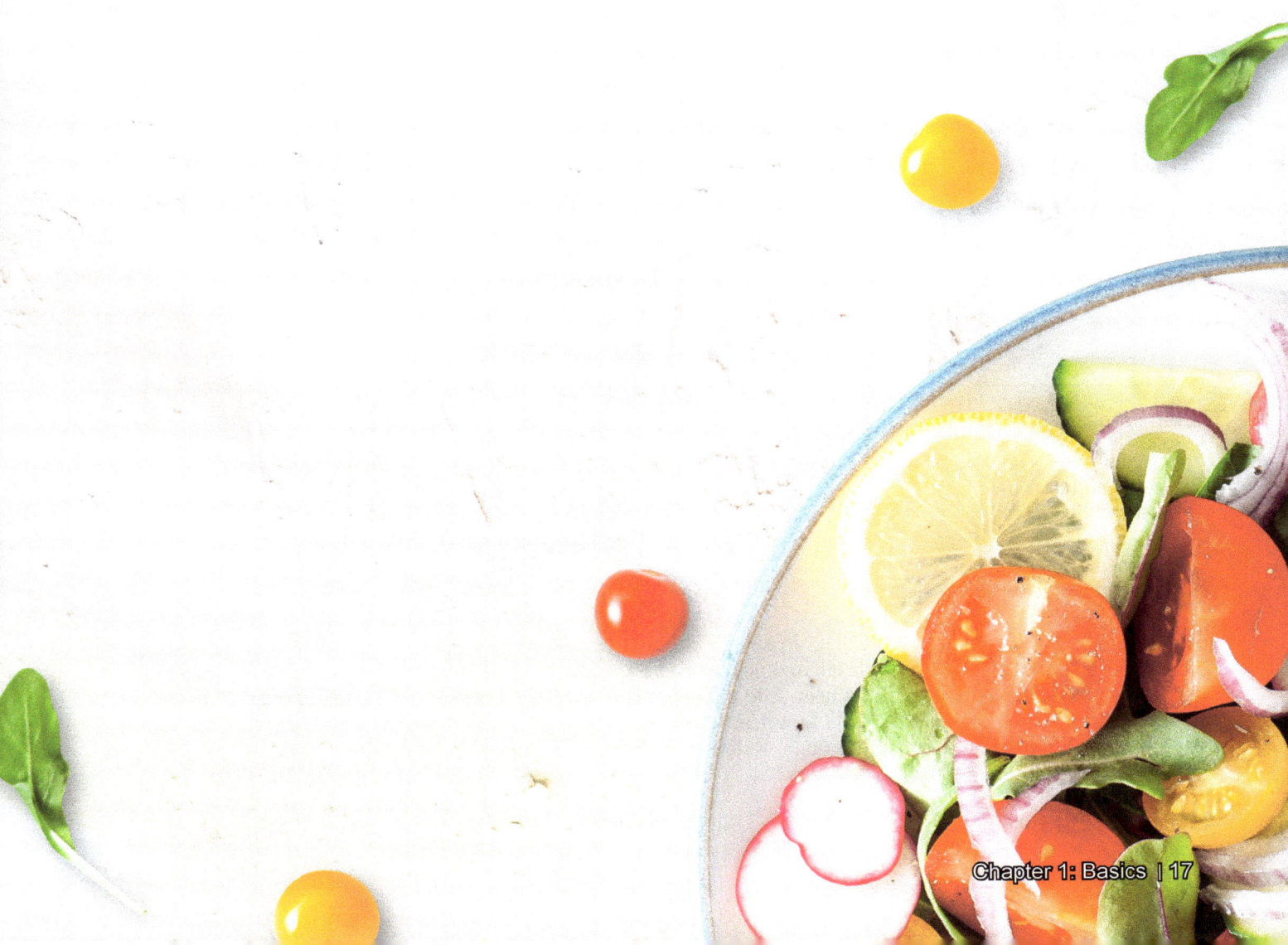

Baked Fish with Olives

Prep time: 10 minutes | Cook time: 12 minutes | Serves 4

2 tablespoons olive oil
2 shallots, diced
1 (28 ounces / 794 g) can diced tomatoes, drained
Freshly ground black pepper
½ cup chopped pitted kalamata olives
¼ cup chopped fresh Italian parsley (optional)

½ onion, chopped
4 garlic cloves, minced
Sea salt
1 pound (454 g) cod or other white-fleshed fish
¼ cup crumbled feta cheese, for topping

1. Preheat the oven to 375°F (191°C). 2. In a large oven-safe skillet, heat the olive oil over medium-high heat. Add the onion, shallots, and garlic and sauté for 5 to 6 minutes, until softened. Add the tomatoes and season with salt and pepper. Cook, stirring occasionally, for 4 minutes. 3. Place the fish on top of the tomato mixture and evenly sprinkle with the olives and feta. Transfer the skillet to the oven and bake for 15 to 20 minutes, until the fish is cooked through. 4. Garnish with the parsley, if desired, and serve.

Per Serving
Calories: 229 | Total fat: 12g | Total carbs: 12g | Sugar: 6g | Protein: 21g | Fiber: 5g | Sodium: 724mg

Pan-Seared Shrimp Skewers

Prep time: 20 minutes | Cook time: 6 minutes | Serves 4

¼ cup olive oil
1 tablespoon dried oregano
Sea salt
1 pound (454 g) medium shrimp (36/40 count), peeled and deveined

Zest and juice of 1 lemon
¼ teaspoon red pepper flakes (optional)
Freshly ground black pepper

1. In a large bowl, stir together the olive oil, lemon zest, oregano, and red pepper flakes, if desired. Season with salt and black pepper. Add the shrimp and mix well. Cover the bowl with plastic wrap and refrigerate for 15 minutes. 2. Remove the bowl from the refrigerator and thread the shrimp onto skewers. Discard any remaining marinade. 3. Heat a large skillet over medium heat. Place the skewers in the skillet and sear the shrimp for 3 to 4 minutes per side, until just cooked through. 4. Drizzle with the lemon juice and serve.

Per Serving
Calories: 204 | Total fat: 15g | Total carbs: 2g | Sugar: 0g | Protein: 15g | Fiber: 0g | Sodium: 581mg

Shrimp Saganaki

Prep time: 15 minutes | Cook time: 15 minutes | Serves 4

1 pound (454 g) medium shrimp (36/40 count), peeled and deveined
Zest of 1 lemon
Sea salt
½ cup chopped onion
½ cup crumbled feta cheese

½ cup plus 1 tablespoon olive oil, divided
½ cup white wine
2 garlic cloves, minced
Freshly ground black pepper
1 tomato, diced
¼ cup chopped fresh Italian parsley

1. Preheat the oven to 400°F (204°C). 2. In a large bowl, stir together the shrimp, ½ cup of olive oil, the wine, lemon zest, and garlic. Season with salt and pepper and set aside. 3. In a Dutch oven, heat the remaining 1 tablespoon of olive oil over medium heat. Add the onion and sauté for 5 minutes, or until softened. Add the tomato and the shrimp mixture and cook for 3 minutes. 4. Transfer the Dutch oven to the oven and bake for 7 minutes, or until the shrimp are just cooked through. Remove from the oven, top with the feta, and bake for 1 to 2 minutes more. 5. Garnish with the parsley and serve.

Per Serving
Calories: 321 | Total fat: 22g | Total carbs: 6g | Sugar: 3g | Protein: 19g | Fiber: 1g | Sodium: 759mg

Cod and Potatoes in Avgolemono

Prep time: 10 minutes | Cook time: 25 minutes | Serves 4

4 cups chicken broth
¼ cup chopped onion
Sea salt
4 (5 ounces / 142-g) cod fillets
Juice of 1 lemon

1 pound (454 g) baby red potatoes, quartered
3 garlic cloves, minced
Freshly ground black pepper
2 large eggs

1. In a large stockpot, bring the broth to a boil over high heat. Add the potatoes, onion, and garlic. Season with salt and pepper, cover, reduce the heat to low, and simmer for 15 minutes. Add the cod and simmer for 7 to 10 minutes more, until the fish is cooked through. 2. While the cod is simmering, in a small bowl, whisk together the eggs and lemon juice. While whisking continuously, slowly add 1 cup of the hot broth to the bowl with the egg mixture and whisk for a few seconds more to temper the egg mixture. Pour the mixture from the bowl back into the stockpot and stir to combine. Serve.

Per Serving
Calories: 241 | Total fat: 4g | Total carbs: 21g | Sugar: 2g | Protein: 30g | Fiber: 2g | Sodium: 172mg

Tomato and White Beans with Garlic Shrimp

Prep time: 10 minutes | Cook time: 10 minutes | Serves 4

3 tablespoons olive oil
4 garlic cloves, minced
2 (15 ounces / 425-g) cans white beans, drained and rinsed
1 pound (454 g) medium shrimp (36/40 count), peeled and deveined

½ onion, diced
1 (15 ounces / 425-g) can diced tomatoes, with their juices
½ to ¾ cup water
¼ cup chopped fresh Italian parsley

1. In a large skillet, heat the olive oil over medium-high heat. Add the onion and garlic and sauté for 4 minutes. Add the tomatoes and cook for 2 minutes. Add the beans and water and bring to a simmer. 2. Add the shrimp and simmer for 3 to 4 minutes, until the shrimp are just cooked through. 3. Serve garnished with the parsley.

Per Serving
Calories: 385 | Total fat: 12g | Total carbs: 41g | Sugar: 4g | Protein: 30g | Fiber: 11g | Sodium: 676mg

Foil-Baked Fish

Prep time: 10 minutes | Cook time: 20 minutes | Serves 4

4 (5 ounces / 142 g) cod or other white-fleshed fish fillets
1 tablespoon freshly squeezed lemon juice
Freshly ground black pepper

2 to 3 tablespoons olive oil
2 to 3 garlic cloves, minced
Sea salt

1. Preheat the oven to 400°F (204°C). Cut four 12-inch squares of aluminum foil and lay them on a clean work surface. 2. Pat the fish dry with paper towels and place one fillet on each sheet of foil. 3. In a small bowl, mix the olive oil, garlic, and lemon juice and season with salt and pepper. Brush the oil mixture over both sides of the fish. Fold the foil over the fish to enclose it and crimp the edges of the foil to seal. 4. Place the foil packets on a baking sheet and bake for 15 to 20 minutes, until the fish is cooked through and flakes easily with a fork. 5. Remove from the oven and serve. Be sure to tell your guests to be careful of the hot steam when opening their packets.

Per Serving:
Calories: 179 | Total fat: 8g | Total carbs: 1g | Sugar: 1g | Protein: 25g | Fiber: 1g | Sodium: 116mg

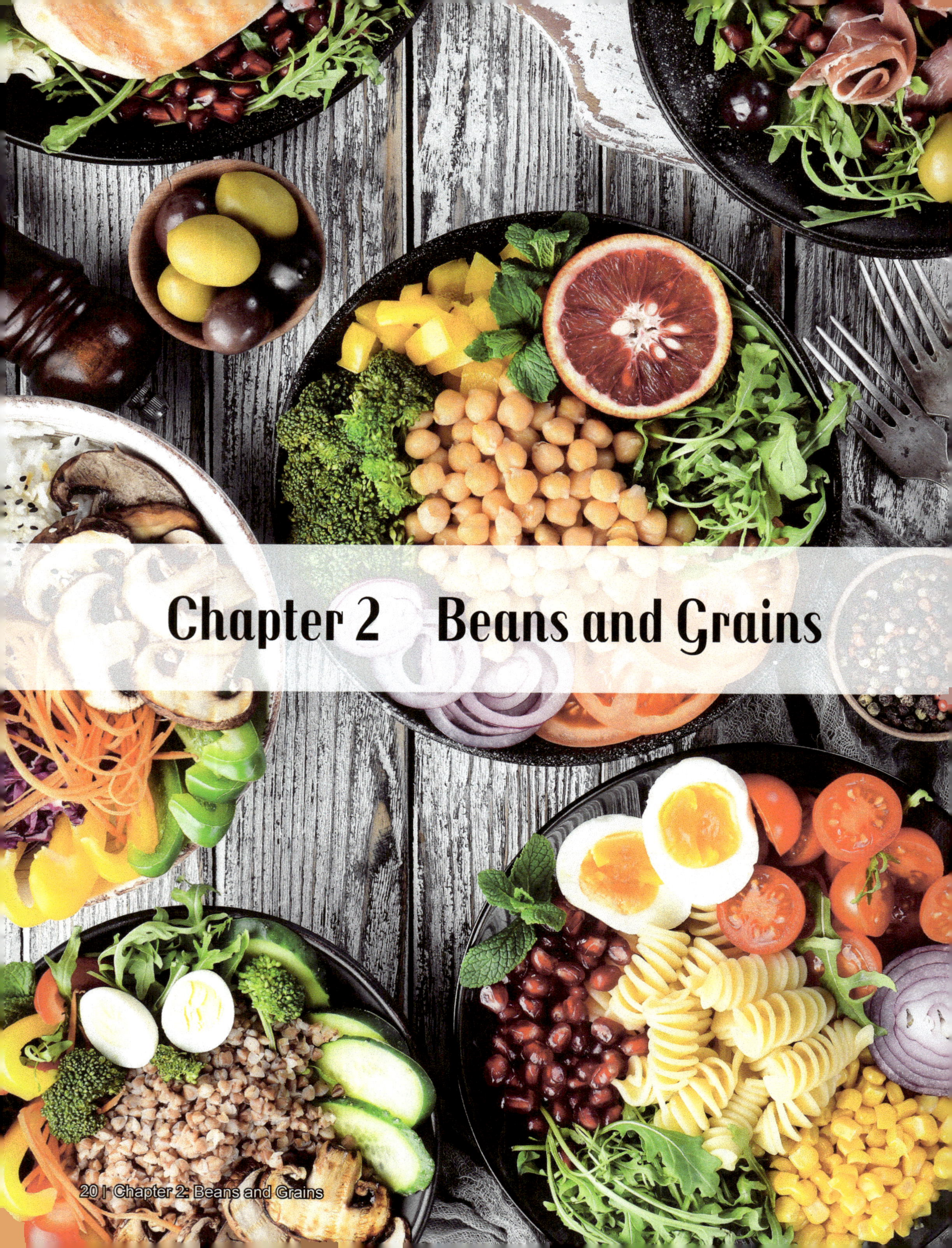

Chapter 2   Beans and Grains

7   **Barley Salad with Lemon-Tahini Dressing**   22
8   **Buckwheat Bake with Root Vegetables**   22
9   **Herbed Polenta**   23
10 **Moroccan Date Pilaf**   23
11 **Farro Salad with Tomatoes and Olives**   23
12 **Earthy Lentil and Rice Pilaf**   24
13 **Rice with Pork Chops**   24
14 **Barley Risotto**   24
15 **Three-Bean Salad**   25
16 **Vegetarian Dinner Loaf**   25
17 **Amaranth Salad**   26
18 **White Bean Soup with Kale and Lemon**   26
19 **Garlic Shrimp with Quinoa**   26
20 **Spanish Rice**   27
21 **Revithosoupa (Chickpea Soup)**   27
22 **Mediterranean Creamed Green Peas**   27
23 **Three-Grain Pilaf**   28
24 **Harissa Rice with White Beans**   28
25 **Farro and Mushroom Risotto**   28
26 **Two-Bean Bulgur Chili**   29

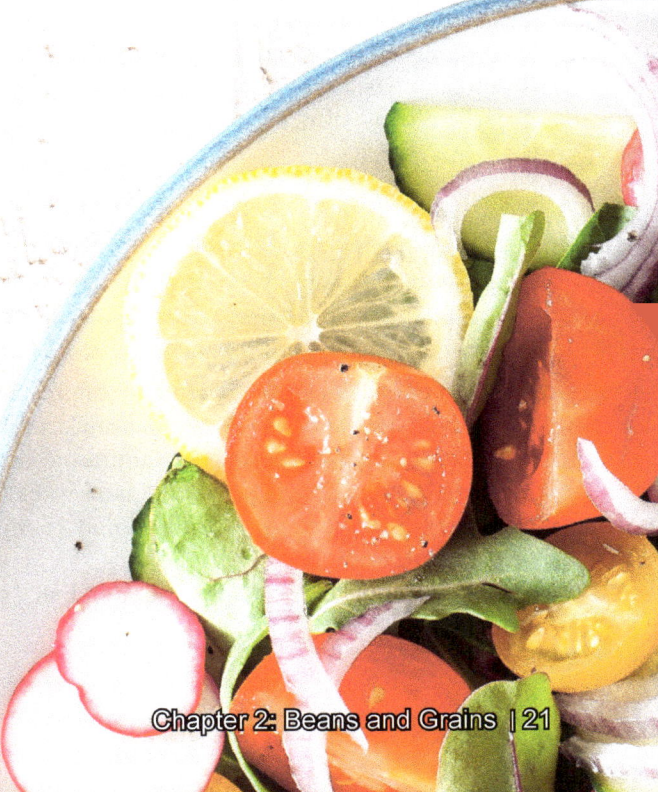

Barley Salad with Lemon-Tahini Dressing

Prep time: 15 minutes | Cook time: 10 minutes | Serves 4 to 6

1½ cups pearl barley
1½ teaspoons table salt, for cooking barley
1 teaspoon grated lemon zest plus
¼ cup juice (2 lemons)
¾ teaspoon table salt
1 carrot, peeled and shredded
4 scallions, sliced thin
¼ cup coarsely chopped fresh mint

5 tablespoons extra-virgin olive oil, divided
¼ cup tahini
1 tablespoon sumac, divided
1 garlic clove, minced
1 English cucumber, cut into ½-inch pieces
1 red bell pepper, stemmed, seeded, and chopped
2 tablespoons finely chopped jarred hot cherry peppers

1. Combine 6 cups water, barley, 1 tablespoon oil, and 1½ teaspoons salt in Instant Pot. Lock lid in place and close pressure release valve. Select high pressure cook function and cook for 8 minutes. Turn off Instant Pot and let pressure release naturally for 15 minutes. Quick-release any remaining pressure, then carefully remove lid, allowing steam to escape away from you. Drain barley, spread onto rimmed baking sheet, and let cool completely, about 15 minutes. 2. Meanwhile, whisk remaining ¼ cup oil, tahini, 2 tablespoons water, lemon zest and juice, 1 teaspoon sumac, garlic, and ¾ teaspoon salt in large bowl until combined; let sit for 15 minutes. 3. Measure out and reserve ½ cup dressing for serving. Add barley, cucumber, carrot, bell pepper, scallions, and cherry peppers to bowl with dressing and gently toss to combine. Season with salt and pepper to taste. Transfer salad to serving dish and sprinkle with mint and remaining 2 teaspoons sumac. Serve, passing reserved dressing separately.

Per Serving
Cal: 370 | Total Fat: 18g | Sat Fat: 2.5g | Chol: 0mg | Sodium: 510mg | Total Carbs: 47g, Fiber: 10g, Total Sugar: 3g | Added Sugar: 0g | Protein: 8g

Buckwheat Bake with Root Vegetables

Prep time: 15 minutes | Cook time: 30 minutes | Serves 6

Olive oil cooking spray
2 carrots, sliced
2 celery stalks, chopped
¼ cup plus 1 tablespoon olive oil, divided
1 cup buckwheat groats
2 garlic cloves, minced
1 teaspoon salt

2 large potatoes, cubed
1 small rutabaga, cubed
½ teaspoon smoked paprika
2 rosemary sprigs
2 cups vegetable broth
½ yellow onion, chopped

1. Preheat the air fryer to 380°F (193°C). Lightly coat the inside of a 5-cup capacity casserole dish with olive oil cooking spray. (The shape of the casserole dish will depend upon the size of the air fryer, but it needs to be able to hold at least 5 cups.) 2. In a large bowl, toss the potatoes, carrots, rutabaga, and celery with the paprika and ¼ cup olive oil. 3. Pour the vegetable mixture into the prepared casserole dish and top with the rosemary sprigs. Place the casserole dish into the air fryer and bake for 15 minutes. 4. While the vegetables are cooking, rinse and drain the buckwheat groats. 5. In a medium saucepan over medium-high heat, combine the groats, vegetable broth, garlic, onion, and salt with the remaining 1 tablespoon olive oil. Bring the mixture to a boil, then reduce the heat to low, cover, and cook for 10 to 12 minutes. 6. Remove the casserole dish from the air fryer. Remove the rosemary sprigs and discard. Pour the cooked buckwheat into the dish with the vegetables and stir to combine. Cover with aluminum foil and bake for an additional 15 minutes. 7. Stir before serving.

Per Serving
Calories: 344 | Total Fat: 13g | Saturated Fat: 2g | Protein: 8g | Total Carbohydrates: 50g | Fiber: 8g | Sugar: 4g | Cholesterol: 0mg

Herbed Polenta

Prep time: 10 minutes | Cook time: 3 to 5 hours | Serves 4

- 1 cup stone-ground polenta
- 1 tablespoon extra-virgin olive oil
- 1 small onion, minced
- 1 teaspoon sea salt
- 1 teaspoon dried oregano
- ½ teaspoon freshly ground black pepper
- 4 cups low-sodium vegetable stock or low-sodium chicken stock
- 2 garlic cloves, minced
- 1 teaspoon dried parsley
- 1 teaspoon dried thyme
- ½ cup grated Parmesan cheese

1. In a slow cooker, combine the polenta, vegetable stock, olive oil, onion, garlic, salt, parsley, oregano, thyme, and pepper. Stir to mix well. 2. Cover the cooker and cook for 3 to 5 hours on Low heat. 3. Stir in the Parmesan cheese for serving.

Per Serving

Calories: 244 | Total fat: 7g | Sodium: 956mg | Carbohydrates: 33g | Fiber: 4g | Sugar: 3g | Protein: 9g

Moroccan Date Pilaf

Prep time: 10 minutes | Cook time: 30 minutes | Serves 4

- 3 tablespoons olive oil
- 3 garlic cloves, minced
- ½ to 1 tablespoon harissa
- ¼ cup dried cranberries
- ¼ teaspoon ground cinnamon
- ¼ teaspoon sea salt
- 2 cups chicken broth
- 1 onion, chopped
- 1 cup uncooked long-grain rice
- 5 or 6 Medjool dates (or another variety), pitted and chopped
- ½ teaspoon ground turmeric
- ¼ teaspoon freshly ground black pepper
- ¼ cup shelled whole pistachios, for garnish

1. In a large stockpot, heat the olive oil over medium heat. Add the onion and garlic and sauté for 3 to 5 minutes, until the onion is soft. Add the rice and cook for 3 minutes, until the grains start to turn opaque. Add the harissa, dates, cranberries, cinnamon, turmeric, salt, and pepper and cook for 30 seconds. Add the broth and bring to a boil, then reduce the heat to low, cover, and simmer for 20 minutes, or until the liquid has been absorbed. 2. Remove the rice from the heat and stir in the nuts. Let stand for 10 minutes before serving.

Per Serving

Calories: 368 | Total fat: 15g | Total carbs: 54g | Sugar: 13g | Protein: 6g | Fiber: 4g | Sodium: 83mg

Farro Salad with Tomatoes and Olives

Prep time: 10 minutes | Cook time: 20 minutes | Serves 6

- 10 ounces (283 g) farro, rinsed and drained
- 4 Roma tomatoes, seeded and chopped
- ½ cup sliced black olives
- ¼ cup extra-virgin olive oil
- ¼ teaspoon ground black pepper
- 4 cups water
- 4 scallions, green parts only, thinly sliced
- ¼ cup minced fresh flat-leaf parsley
- 2 tablespoons balsamic vinegar

1. Place farro and water in the Instant Pot®. Close lid and set steam release to Sealing. Press the Multigrain button and set time to 20 minutes. When the timer beeps, let pressure release naturally, about 30 minutes. 2. Open lid and fluff with a fork. Transfer to a bowl and cool 30 minutes. Add tomatoes, scallions, black olives, and parsley and mix well. 3. In a small bowl, whisk together oil, balsamic vinegar, and pepper. Pour over salad and toss to evenly coat. Refrigerate for at least 4 hours before serving. Serve chilled or at room temperature.

Per Serving

Calories: 288 | Fat: 14g | Protein: 7g | Sodium: 159mg | Fiber: 3 | Carbohydrates: 31g | Sugar: 4g

Earthy Lentil and Rice Pilaf

Prep time: 5 minutes | Cook time: 50 minutes | Serves 6

¼ cup extra-virgin olive oil
6 cups water
1 teaspoon salt
1 cup basmati rice

1 large onion, chopped
1 teaspoon ground cumin
2 cups brown lentils, picked over and rinsed

1. In a medium pot over medium heat, cook the olive oil and onions for 7 to 10 minutes until the edges are browned. 2. Turn the heat to high, add the water, cumin, and salt, and bring this mixture to a boil, boiling for about 3 minutes. 3. Add the lentils and turn the heat to medium-low. Cover the pot and cook for 20 minutes, stirring occasionally. 4. Stir in the rice and cover; cook for an additional 20 minutes. 5. Fluff the rice with a fork and serve warm.

Per Serving
Calories: 397 | Protein: 18g | Total Carbohydrates: 60g | Sugars: 4g | Fiber: 18g | Total Fat: 11g | Saturated Fat: 1g | Cholesterol: 0mg | Sodium: 396mg

Rice with Pork Chops

Prep time: 10 minutes | Cook time: 3 to 5 hours | Serves 4

1 cup raw long-grain brown rice, rinsed
1 cup sliced tomato
1 small onion, chopped
2 teaspoons dried oregano
1 teaspoon sea salt
4 thick-cut pork chops

2½ cups low-sodium chicken broth
8 ounces (227 g) fresh spinach, chopped
2 garlic cloves, minced
2 teaspoons dried basil
½ teaspoon freshly ground black pepper
¼ cup grated Parmesan cheese

1. In a slow cooker, combine the rice, chicken broth, tomato, spinach, onion, garlic, oregano, basil, salt, and pepper. Stir to mix well. 2. Place the pork chops on top of the rice mixture. 3. Cover the cooker and cook for 3 to 5 hours on Low heat. 4. Top with the Parmesan cheese for serving.

Per Serving
Calories: 375 | Total fat: 10g | Sodium: 1,042mg | Carbohydrates: 43g | Fiber: 6g | Sugar: 1g | Protein: 31g

Barley Risotto

Prep time: 10 minutes | Cook time: 30 minutes | Serves 6

2 tablespoons olive oil
1 clove garlic, peeled and minced
1½ cups pearl barley, rinsed and drained
4 cups low-sodium chicken broth
1 cup grated Parmesan cheese
¼ teaspoon salt

1 large onion, peeled and diced
1 stalk celery, finely minced
⅓ cup dried mushrooms
2¼ cups water
2 tablespoons minced fresh parsley

1. Press the Sauté button on the Instant Pot® and heat oil. Add onion and sauté 5 minutes. Add garlic and cook 30 seconds. Stir in celery, barley, mushrooms, broth, and water. Press the Cancel button. 2. Close lid, set steam release to Sealing, press the Manual button, and set time to 18 minutes. When the timer beeps, quick-release the pressure until the float valve drops and open the lid. 3. Drain off excess liquid, leaving enough to leave the risotto slightly soupy. Press the Cancel button, then press the Sauté button and cook until thickened, about 5 minutes. Stir in cheese, parsley, and salt. Serve immediately.

Per Serving
Calories: 175 | Fat: 9g | Protein: 10g | Sodium: 447mg | Fiber: 2g | Carbohydrates: 13g | Sugar: 2g

Three-Bean Salad

Prep time: 15 minutes | Cook time: 30 minutes | Serves 8

- ¼ pound (113 g) dried pinto beans, soaked overnight and drained
- ¼ pound (113 g) dried red beans, soaked overnight and drained
- 1 stalk celery, chopped
- ½ medium green bell pepper, seeded and chopped
- ¼ cup minced fresh flat-leaf parsley
- 3 tablespoons red wine vinegar
- ½ teaspoon ground black pepper
- ¼ pound (113 g) dried black beans, soaked overnight and drained
- 8 cups water
- 1 tablespoon light olive oil
- ½ medium red onion, peeled and chopped
- ¼ cup minced fresh cilantro
- 3 tablespoons extra-virgin olive oil
- 1 tablespoon honey
- ½ teaspoon sea salt

1. Place beans, water, and light olive oil in the Instant Pot®. Close lid, set steam release to Sealing, and press the Bean button and cook for the default time of 30 minutes. When the timer beeps, let pressure release naturally, about 20 minutes. Open lid and drain beans. Cool to room temperature. 2. Transfer cooled beans to a large bowl. Add celery, onion, bell pepper, cilantro, and parsley. Mix well. In a small bowl, whisk together extra-virgin olive oil, vinegar, honey, black pepper, and salt. Pour dressing over bean mixture and toss to coat. Refrigerate for 4 hours before serving.

Per Serving

Calories: 208 | Fat: 8g | Protein: 8g | Sodium: 162mg | Fiber: 6 | Carbohydrates: 26g | Sugar: 3g

Vegetarian Dinner Loaf

Prep time: 10 minutes | Cook time: 45 minutes | Serves 6

- 1 cup dried pinto beans, soaked overnight and drained
- 1 tablespoon vegetable oil
- 1 cup diced onion
- 1 cup chopped walnuts
- 1 large egg, beaten
- 1 teaspoon garlic powder
- 1 teaspoon dried parsley
- ½ teaspoon ground black pepper
- 8 cups water, divided
- 1 teaspoon salt
- ½ cup rolled oats
- ¾ cup ketchup
- 1 teaspoon dried basil
- ½ teaspoon salt

1. Add beans and 4 cups water to the Instant Pot®. Close lid, set steam release to Sealing, press the Manual button, and set time to 1 minute. When the timer beeps, quick-release the pressure until the float valve drops. Press the Cancel button. 2. Open lid, then drain and rinse beans and return to the pot with remaining 4 cups water. Soak for 1 hour. 3. Preheat oven to 350°F (177°C). 4. Add the oil and salt to pot. Close lid, set steam release to Sealing, press the Manual button, and set time to 11 minutes. When the timer beeps, let pressure release naturally, about 25 minutes, and open lid. Drain beans and pour into a large mixing bowl. 5. Stir in onion, walnuts, oats, egg, ketchup, garlic powder, basil, parsley, salt, and pepper. Spread the mixture into a loaf pan and bake for 30–35 minutes. Cool for 20 minutes in pan before slicing and serving.

Per Serving

Calories: 278 | Fat: 17g | Protein: 9g | Sodium: 477mg | Fiber: 6 | Carbohydrates: 27g | Sugar: 8g

Amaranth Salad

Prep time: 5 minutes | Cook time: 6 minutes | Serves 4

2 cups water
1 teaspoon dried Greek oregano
½ teaspoon ground black pepper
2 teaspoons red wine vinegar

1 cup amaranth
½ teaspoon salt
1 tablespoon extra-virgin olive oil

1. Add water and amaranth to the Instant Pot®. Close lid, set steam release to Sealing, press the Manual button, and set time to 6 minutes. When the timer beeps, quick-release the pressure until the float valve drops. 2. Open lid and fluff amaranth with a fork. Add oregano, salt, and pepper. Mix well. Drizzle with olive oil and wine vinegar. Serve hot.

Per Serving
Calories: 93 | Fat: 5g | Protein: 3g | Sodium: 299mg | Fiber: 3 | Carbohydrates: 12g | Sugar: 0g

White Bean Soup with Kale and Lemon

Prep time: 15 minutes | Cook time: 27 minutes | Serves 8

1 tablespoon light olive oil
1 medium yellow onion, peeled and chopped
1 tablespoon chopped fresh oregano
1 pound (454 g) dried Great Northern beans, soaked overnight and drained
1 tablespoon extra-virgin olive oil

2 stalks celery, chopped
2 cloves garlic, peeled and minced
4 cups chopped kale
8 cups vegetable broth
¼ cup lemon juice
1 teaspoon ground black pepper

1. Press the Sauté button on the Instant Pot® and heat light olive oil. Add celery and onion and cook 5 minutes. Add garlic and oregano and sauté 30 seconds. Add kale and turn to coat, then cook until just starting to wilt, about 1 minute. Press the Cancel button. 2. Add beans, broth, lemon juice, extra-virgin olive oil, and pepper to the Instant Pot® and stir well. Close lid, set steam release to Sealing, press the Manual button, and set time to 20 minutes. When the timer beeps, let pressure release naturally, about 20 minutes. Open lid and stir well. Serve hot.

Per Serving
Calories: 129 | Fat: 3g | Protein: 7g | Sodium: 501mg | Fiber: 6 | Carbohydrates: 22g | Sugar: 4g

Garlic Shrimp with Quinoa

Prep time: 10 minutes | Cook time: 30 minutes | Serves 4

4 cups chicken broth
5 tablespoons olive oil
6 garlic cloves, minced
1 teaspoon chili powder
Freshly ground black pepper
½ cup crumbled feta cheese, for garnish

2 cups uncooked quinoa, rinsed
½ red onion, chopped
1 tablespoon tomato paste
Sea salt
1½ pounds (680 g) medium shrimp (36/40 count), peeled and deveined

1. In a large stockpot, combine the broth and quinoa and bring to a boil over high heat. Reduce the heat to low, cover, and simmer for 20 to 25 minutes, until the quinoa is cooked. Drain the quinoa and set aside in a medium bowl. 2. Rinse and dry the pot. Pour in the olive oil and heat over medium heat. Add the onion, garlic, tomato paste, and chili powder and cook for 1 minute. Season with salt and pepper and stir to combine. Add the shrimp and cook until the shrimp are pink and just cooked through, 5 to 7 minutes. 3. Return the quinoa to the pot and stir everything together. Remove from the heat. 4. Serve topped with the feta.

Per Serving
Calories: 650 | Total fat: 28g | Total carbs: 62g | Sugar: 2g | Protein: 38g | Fiber: 7g | Sodium: 1,011mg

Spanish Rice

Prep time: 10 minutes | Cook time: 20 minutes | Serves 4

2 tablespoons extra-virgin olive oil
1 large tomato, finely diced
1 teaspoon smoked paprika
1½ cups basmati rice
1 medium onion, finely chopped
2 tablespoons tomato paste
1 teaspoon salt
3 cups water

1. In a medium pot over medium heat, cook the olive oil, onion, and tomato for 3 minutes. 2. Stir in the tomato paste, paprika, salt, and rice. Cook for 1 minute. 3. Add the water, cover the pot, and turn the heat to low. Cook for 12 minutes. 4. Gently toss the rice, cover, and cook for another 3 minutes.

Per Serving
Calories: 328 | Protein: 6g | Total Carbohydrates: 60g | Sugars: 3g | Fiber: 2g | Total Fat: 7g | Saturated Fat: 1g | Cholesterol: 0mg | Sodium: 651mg

Revithosoupa (Chickpea Soup)

Prep time: 10 minutes | Cook time: 30 minutes | Serves 8

1 pound (454 g) dried chickpeas
¾ teaspoon salt
10 strands saffron
1 cup extra-virgin olive oil
3 tablespoons lemon juice
4 cups water
½ teaspoon ground black pepper
2 medium onions, peeled and diced
1 teaspoon dried oregano
2 tablespoons chopped fresh parsley

1. Add chickpeas, water, salt, pepper, saffron, onions, oil, and oregano to the Instant Pot® and stir well. Close lid, set steam release to Sealing, press the Bean button, and cook for the default time of 30 minutes. 2. When the timer beeps, let pressure release naturally, about 25 minutes. Open lid. Serve hot or cold, sprinkled with lemon juice. Garnish with chopped parsley.

Per Serving
Calories: 464 | Fat: 30g | Protein: 12g | Sodium: 236mg | Fiber: 10g | Carbohydrates: 38g | Sugar: 8g

Mediterranean Creamed Green Peas

Prep time: 5 minutes | Cook time: 25 minutes | Serves 4

1 cup cauliflower florets, fresh or frozen
2 tablespoons olive oil
3 cups green peas, fresh or frozen
2 tablespoons fresh thyme leaves, chopped
½ teaspoon salt
Shredded Parmesan cheese, for garnish
½ white onion, roughly chopped
½ cup unsweetened almond milk
3 garlic cloves, minced
1 teaspoon fresh rosemary leaves, chopped
½ teaspoon black pepper
Fresh parsley, for garnish

1. Preheat the air fryer to 380°F (193°C). 2. In a large bowl, combine the cauliflower florets and onion with the olive oil and toss well to coat. 3. Put the cauliflower-and-onion mixture into the air fryer basket in an even layer and bake for 15 minutes. 4. Transfer the cauliflower and onion to a food processor. Add the almond milk and pulse until smooth. 5. In a medium saucepan, combine the cauliflower puree, peas, garlic, thyme, rosemary, salt, and pepper and mix well. Cook over medium heat for an additional 10 minutes, stirring regularly. 6. Serve with a sprinkle of Parmesan cheese and chopped fresh parsley.

Per Serving
Calories: 87 | Total Fat: 4g | Saturated Fat: 1g | Protein: 4g | Total Carbohydrates: 10g | Fiber: 3g | Sugar: 4g | Cholesterol: 0mg

Three-Grain Pilaf

Prep time: 10 minutes | Cook time: 10 minutes | Serves 6

2 tablespoons extra-virgin olive oil
1 cup jasmine rice
½ cup quinoa, rinsed and drained
¼ teaspoon salt
½ cup sliced scallions
½ cup millet
2½ cups vegetable stock
¼ teaspoon ground black pepper

1. Press the Sauté button on the Instant Pot® and heat oil. Add scallions and cook until just tender, 2 minutes. Add rice, millet, and quinoa and cook for 3 minutes to toast. Add stock and stir well. Press the Cancel button. 2. Close lid, set steam release to Sealing, press the Manual button, and set time to 4 minutes. When the timer beeps, quick-release the pressure until the float valve drops and open the lid. Fluff pilaf with a fork and stir in salt and pepper. Serve warm.

Per Serving
Calories: 346 | Fat: 7g | Protein: 8g | Sodium: 341mg | Fiber: 4g | Carbohydrates: 61g | Sugar: 1g

Harissa Rice with White Beans

Prep time: 5 minutes | Cook time: 30 minutes | Serves 4

1 tablespoon olive oil
1 tablespoon harissa
1 (15 ounces / 425-g) can great northern beans, drained and rinsed
1 cup uncooked white rice
2 garlic cloves, minced
2 cups vegetable broth
¼ teaspoon sea salt

1. In a large stockpot, heat the olive oil over medium-high heat. Add the rice and sauté for 2 to 3 minutes. Add the harissa and garlic and sauté for 1 to 2 minutes. Add the beans and cook for 1 minute. 2. Add the broth and salt, increase the heat to high, and bring to a boil. Boil for 1 minute, then reduce the heat to low, cover, and simmer for 20 minutes, or until the liquid has been absorbed. Serve.

Per Serving
Calories: 295 | Total fat: 4g | Total carbs: 55g | Sugar: 1g | Protein: 9g | Fiber: 6g | Sodium: 355mg

Farro and Mushroom Risotto

Prep time: 10 minutes | Cook time: 20 minutes | Serves 6

2 tablespoons olive oil
16 ounces (454 g) sliced button mushrooms
½ teaspoon ground black pepper
½ teaspoon dried oregano
1 cup farro, rinsed and drained
¼ cup grated Parmesan cheese
1 medium yellow onion, peeled and diced
½ teaspoon salt
½ teaspoon dried thyme
1 clove garlic, peeled and minced
1½ cups vegetable broth
2 tablespoons minced fresh flat-leaf parsley

1. Press the Sauté button on the Instant Pot® and heat oil. Add onion and mushrooms and sauté 8 minutes. Add salt, pepper, thyme, and oregano and cook 30 seconds. Add garlic and cook for 30 seconds. Press the Cancel button. 2. Stir in farro and broth. Close lid, set steam release to Sealing, press the Manual button, and set time to 10 minutes. When timer beeps, let pressure release naturally for 10 minutes, then quick-release the remaining pressure until the float valve drops. 3 Top with cheese and parsley before serving.

Per Serving
Calories: 215 | Fat: 8g | Protein: 11g | Sodium: 419mg | Fiber: 3g | Carbohydrates: 24g | Sugar: 2g

Two-Bean Bulgur Chili

Prep time: 10 minutes | Cook time: 30 minutes | Serves 4 to 5

2 tablespoons olive oil
2 celery stalks, diced
1 jalapeño pepper, seeded and chopped
1 (28 ounces / 794 g) can diced tomatoes
1½ teaspoons chili powder
2 teaspoons ground cumin
1 (15 ounces / 425-g) can cannellini beans, drained and rinsed
4 cups chicken broth
Freshly ground black pepper
1 onion, diced
1 carrot, diced
3 garlic cloves, minced
1 tablespoon tomato paste
2 teaspoons dried oregano
1 (15 ounces / 425-g) can black beans, drained and rinsed
¾ cup dried bulgur
Sea salt

1. In a Dutch oven, heat the olive oil over medium-high heat. Add the onion, celery, carrot, jalapeño, and garlic and sauté until the vegetables are tender, about 4 minutes. 2. Reduce the heat to medium and add the diced tomatoes, tomato paste, chili powder, oregano, and cumin. Cook for 3 minutes, then add the black beans, cannellini beans, bulgur, and broth. 3. Increase the heat to high, cover, and bring to a boil. Reduce the heat to low and simmer until the chili is cooked to your desired thickness, about 30 minutes. Season with salt and black pepper and serve.

Per Serving
Calories: 385 | Total fat: 9g | Total carbs: 64g | Sugar: 8g | Protein: 17g | Fiber: 20g | Sodium: 325mg

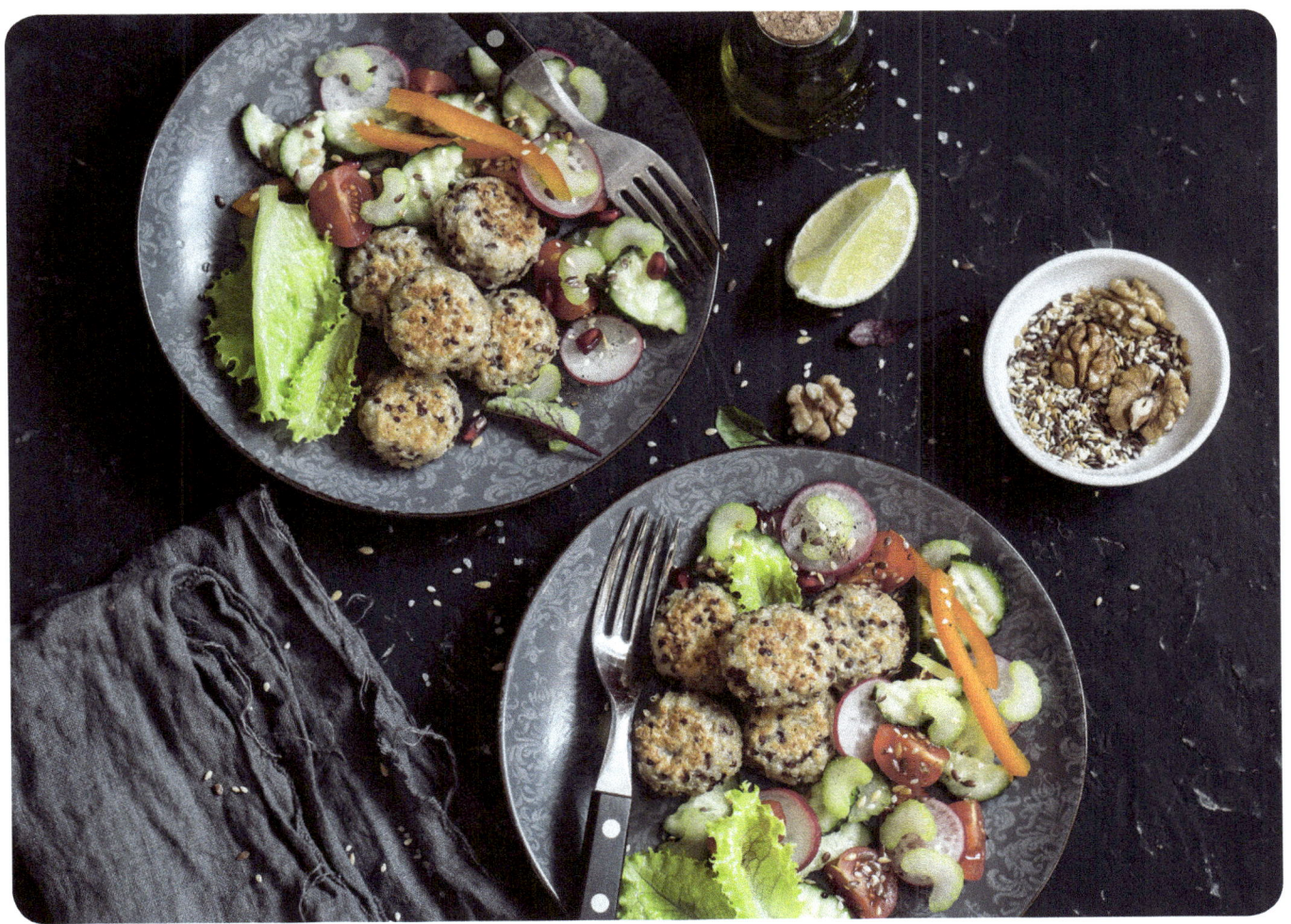

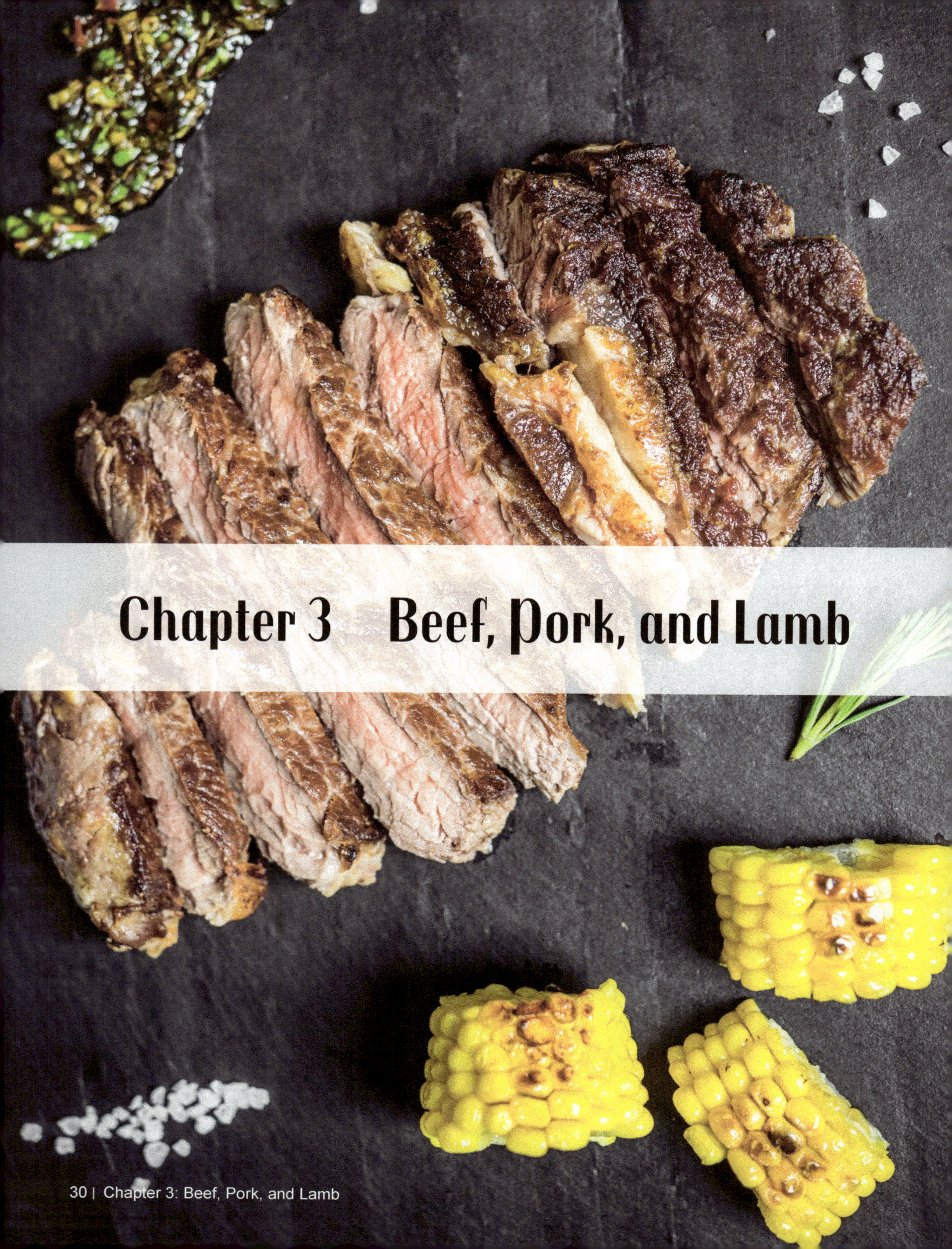

Chapter 3   Beef, Pork, and Lamb

27 **Pork with Orzo**   32
28 **Spiced Oven-Baked Meatballs with Tomato Sauce**   32
29 **Spicy Lamb Burgers with Harissa Mayo**   33
30 **Meatballs in Creamy Almond Sauce**   33
31 **Tahini Beef and Potatoes**   34
32 **Pork Sausage with White Beans and Mustard Greens**   34
33 **Easy Honey-Garlic Pork Chops**   35
34 **Wine-Braised Short Ribs with Potatoes**   35
35 **Greek Lamb Chops**   36
36 **Beef and Goat Cheese Stuffed Peppers**   36
37 **Greek Lamb Burgers**   36
38 **Balsamic Pork Chops with Figs and Pears**   37
39 **Lamb Kofta**   37
40 **Pork Casserole with Fennel and Potatoes**   37
41 **Pork Tenderloin with Vegetable Ragu**   38
42 **Hearty Stewed Beef in Tomato Sauce**   38
43 **Giouvarlakia Soup**   39
44 **Beef Meatballs in Garlic Cream Sauce**   39

Pork with Orzo

Prep time: 10 minutes | Cook time: 30 minutes | Serves 4

2 tablespoons olive oil
2 carrots, chopped
2 garlic cloves, minced
1 teaspoon Italian seasoning
2 cups chicken broth
2 cups arugula
Freshly ground black pepper
2 yellow squash, diced
½ red onion, chopped
1 pound (454 g) boneless pork loin chops, cut into 2-inch pieces
1 cup dried orzo
Sea salt
Grated Parmesan cheese (optional)

1. In a Dutch oven, heat the olive oil over medium-high heat. Add the squash, carrots, onion, and garlic and sauté for 5 minutes, or until softened. Add the pork and Italian seasoning and sauté, stirring occasionally, for 3 to 5 minutes, until browned. 2. Increase the heat to high, add the broth, and bring to a boil. Add the orzo, reduce the heat to medium-low, and simmer, stirring occasionally, for 8 minutes. Add the arugula and stir until wilted. Turn off the heat, cover, and let sit for 5 minutes. 3. Season with salt and pepper and serve topped with Parmesan, if desired.

Per Serving
Calories: 423 | Total fat: 11g | Total carbs: 48g | Sugar: 5g | Protein: 31g | Fiber: 4g | Sodium: 127mg

Spiced Oven-Baked Meatballs with Tomato Sauce

Prep time: 25 minutes | Cook time: 1 hour 5 minutes | Serves 4

1 pound (450g) ground chuck
2 garlic cloves, minced
½ teaspoons black pepper
3 tablespoons chopped fresh parsley
3 tablespoons extra virgin olive oil
1 teaspoon red wine vinegar
1 teaspoon fresh lemon juice
3 medium tomatoes, chopped, or
1 (15ounces/425g) can chopped tomatoes
1 teaspoon fine sea salt
¼ teaspoons granulated sugar
¼ cup unseasoned breadcrumbs
1 teaspoon salt
1 teaspoon ground cumin
1 egg, lightly beaten
1 teaspoon tomato paste
2 tablespoons dry red wine
For the sauce
1 tablespoon plus 1 teaspoon tomato paste
¼ cup extra virgin olive oil
¼ teaspoons black pepper
1¾ cups hot water

1. Begin making the meatballs by combining all the ingredients in a large bowl. Knead the mixture for 3 minutes or until all the ingredients are well incorporated. Cover the bowl with plastic wrap and transfer the mixture to the refrigerator to rest for at least 20 minutes. 2. While the meatball mixture is resting, preheat the oven to 350°F (177°C) and begin making the sauce by placing all the ingredients except the hot water in a food processor. Process until smooth and then transfer the mixture to a small pan over medium heat. Add the hot water and mix well. Let the mixture come to a boil and then reduce the heat to low and simmer for 10 minutes. 3. Remove the meatball mixture from the refrigerator and shape it into 24 oblong meatballs. 4. Spread 3 tablespoons of the sauce into the bottom of a large baking dish and place the meatballs in a single layer on top of the sauce. Pour the remaining sauce over the top of the meatballs. 5. Bake for 45 minutes or until the meatballs are lightly brown and then turn the meatballs and bake for an additional 10 minutes. (If the sauce appears to be drying out, add another ¼ cup hot water to the baking dish.) 6. Transfer the meatballs to a serving platter. Spoon the sauce over the meatballs before serving. Store covered in the refrigerator for up to 3 days or in an airtight container in the freezer for up to 3 months.

Per Serving
Calories: 560 | Total fat: 47g | Saturated fat: 13g | Carbohydrate: 12g | Protein: 22g

Spicy Lamb Burgers with Harissa Mayo

Prep timePrep Time: 15 minutes | Cook Time: 10 minutes | Serves 2

½ small onion, minced
2 teaspoons minced fresh parsley
¼ teaspoon salt
1 teaspoon cumin
¼ teaspoon coriander
2 tablespoons olive oil mayonnaise
2 hamburger buns or pitas, fresh greens, tomato slices (optional, for serving)

1 garlic clove, minced
2 teaspoons minced fresh mint
Pinch freshly ground black pepper
1 teaspoon smoked paprika
8 ounces (227 g) lean ground lamb
½ teaspoon harissa paste (more or less to taste)

1. Preheat the grill to medium-high (350–400°F / 177-204°C)) and oil the grill grate. Alternatively, you can cook these in a heavy pan (cast iron is best) on the stovetop. 2. In a large bowl, combine the onion, garlic, parsley, mint, salt, pepper, cumin, paprika, and coriander. Add the lamb and, using your hands, combine the meat with the spices so they are evenly distributed. Form meat mixture into 2 patties. 3. Grill the burgers for 4 minutes per side, or until the internal temperature registers 160°F (71°C) for medium. 4. If cooking on the stovetop, heat the pan to medium-high and oil the pan. Cook the burgers for 5 to 6 minutes per side, or until the internal temperature registers 160°F (71°C). 5. While the burgers are cooking, combine the mayonnaise and harissa in a small bowl. 6. Serve the burgers with the harissa mayonnaise and slices of tomato and fresh greens on a bun or pita—or skip the bun altogether.

Per Serving
Calories: 381 | Total fat: 20g | Total carbs: 27g | Fiber: 2g | Sugar: 4g | Protein: 22g Sodium: 653mg | Cholesterol: 68mg

Meatballs in Creamy Almond Sauce

Prep time: 15 minutes | Cook time: 35 minutes | Serves 4 to 6

8 ounces (227 g) ground veal or pork
½ cup finely minced onion, divided
¼ cup almond flour
1 teaspoon garlic powder
½ teaspoon ground nutmeg
½ cup extra-virgin olive oil, divided
¼ cup slivered almonds
¼ cup unsweetened almond butter

8 ounces (227 g) ground beef
1 large egg, beaten
1½ teaspoons salt, divided
½ teaspoon freshly ground black pepper
2 teaspoons chopped fresh flat-leaf Italian parsley, plus ¼ cup, divided
1 cup dry white wine or chicken broth

1. In a large bowl, combine the veal, beef, ¼ cup onion, and the egg and mix well with a fork. In a small bowl, whisk together the almond flour, 1 teaspoon salt, garlic powder, pepper, and nutmeg. Add to the meat mixture along with 2 teaspoons chopped parsley and incorporate well. Form the mixture into small meatballs, about 1 inch in diameter, and place on a plate. Let sit for 10 minutes at room temperature. 2. In a large skillet, heat ¼ cup oil over medium-high heat. Add the meatballs to the hot oil and brown on all sides, cooking in batches if necessary, 2 to 3 minutes per side. Remove from skillet and keep warm. 3. In the hot skillet, sauté the remaining ¼ cup minced onion in the remaining ¼ cup olive oil for 5 minutes. Reduce the heat to medium-low and add the slivered almonds. Sauté until the almonds are golden, another 3 to 5 minutes. 4. In a small bowl, whisk together the white wine, almond butter, and remaining ½ teaspoon salt. Add to the skillet and bring to a boil, stirring constantly. Reduce the heat to low, return the meatballs to skillet, and cover. Cook until the meatballs are cooked through, another 8 to 10 minutes. 5. Remove from the heat, stir in the remaining ¼ cup chopped parsley, and serve the meatballs warm and drizzled with almond sauce.

Per Serving
Calories: 449 | Total Fat: 42g | Total Carbs: 3g | Net Carbs: 2g | Fiber: 1g | Protein: 16g | Sodium: 696mg

Tahini Beef and Potatoes

Prep time: 10 minutes | Cook time: 30 minutes | Serves 4 to 6

1 pound (454 g) ground beef
½ teaspoon freshly ground black pepper
10 medium golden potatoes
3 cups Greek yogurt
3 cloves garlic, minced

2 teaspoons salt, divided
1 large onion, finely chopped
2 tablespoons extra-virgin olive oil
1 cup tahini
2 cups water

1. Preheat the oven to 450°F (235°C). 2. In a large bowl, using your hands, combine the beef with 1 teaspoon salt, black pepper, and the onion. 3. Form meatballs of medium size (about 1-inch), using about 2 tablespoons of the beef mixture. Place them in a deep 8-by-8-inch casserole dish. 4. Cut the potatoes into ¼-inch-thick slices. Toss them with the olive oil. 5. Lay the potato slices flat on a lined baking sheet. 6. Put the baking sheet with the potatoes and the casserole dish with the meatballs in the oven and bake for 20 minutes. 7. In a large bowl, mix together the yogurt, tahini, garlic, remaining 1 teaspoon salt, and water; set aside. 8. Once you take the meatballs and potatoes out of the oven, use a spatula to transfer the potatoes from the baking sheet to the casserole dish with the meatballs, and leave the beef drippings in the casserole dish for added flavor. 9. Reduce the oven temperature to 375°F (191°C) and pour the yogurt tahini sauce over the beef and potatoes. Return it to the oven for 10 minutes. Once baking is complete, serve warm with a side of rice or pita bread.

Per Serving
Calories: 1,078 | Protein: 58g | Total Carbohydrates: 89g | Sugars: 12g | Fiber: 11g | Total Fat: 59g | Saturated Fat: 14g | Cholesterol: 94mg | Sodium: 1,368mg

Pork Sausage with White Beans and Mustard Greens

Prep time: 15 minutes | Cook time: 20 minutes | Serves 4

2 tablespoons extra-virgin olive oil, divided
1 onion, chopped fine
1 tablespoon minced fresh thyme or 1 teaspoon dried
¾ cup chicken broth
2 (15 ounces / 425-g) cans navy beans, rinsed
½ cup panko bread crumbs
2 tablespoons chopped fresh parsley
4 ounces (113 g) goat cheese, crumbled (1 cup)

1 pound (454 g) hot or sweet Italian sausage (4 sausages)
2 garlic cloves, minced
¼ cup dry white wine
1 pound (454 g) mustard greens, stemmed and cut into 2-inch pieces
½ teaspoon grated lemon zest plus 1 teaspoon juice

1. Using highest sauté function, heat 1 tablespoon oil in Instant Pot for 5 minutes (or until just smoking). Brown sausages on all sides, 6 to 8 minutes; transfer to plate. 2. Add onion to fat left in pot and cook, using highest sauté function, until softened, about 5 minutes. Stir in thyme and garlic and cook until fragrant, about 30 seconds. Stir in broth and wine, scraping up any browned bits, then stir in beans. Add mustard greens, then place sausages on top. Lock lid in place and close pressure release valve. Select high pressure cook function and cook for 2 minutes. 3. Meanwhile, toss panko with remaining 1 tablespoon oil in bowl until evenly coated. Microwave, stirring every 30 seconds, until light golden brown, about 5 minutes. Let cool slightly, then stir in parsley and lemon zest; set aside for serving. 4. Turn off Instant Pot and quick-release pressure. Carefully remove lid, allowing steam to escape away from you. Transfer sausages to plate. Stir lemon juice into bean and mustard greens mixture and season with salt and pepper to taste. Serve sausages with bean and mustard green mixture, sprinkling individual portions with seasoned bread crumbs and goat cheese.

Per Serving
Cal: 520 | Total Fat: 23g | Sat Fat: 9g | Chol: 45mg | Sodium: 1280mg | Total Carbs: 41g, Fiber: 11g | Total Suga;r 5g | Added Sugar 0g | Protein 38g

Easy Honey-Garlic Pork Chops

Prep time: 15 minutes | Cook time: 25 minutes | Serves 4

4 pork chops, boneless or bone-in
⅛ teaspoon freshly ground black pepper
5 tablespoons low-sodium chicken broth, divided
¼ cup honey
¼ teaspoon salt
3 tablespoons extra-virgin olive oil
6 garlic cloves, minced
2 tablespoons apple cider vinegar

1. Season the pork chops with salt and pepper and set aside. 2. In a large sauté pan or skillet, heat the oil over medium-high heat. Add the pork chops and sear for 5 minutes on each side, or until golden brown. 3. Once the searing is complete, move the pork to a dish and reduce the skillet heat from medium-high to medium. Add 3 tablespoons of chicken broth to the pan; this will loosen the bits and flavors from the bottom of the skillet. 4. Once the broth has evaporated, add the garlic to the skillet and cook for 15 to 20 seconds, until fragrant. Add the honey, vinegar, and the remaining 2 tablespoons of broth. Bring the heat back up to medium-high and continue to cook for 3 to 4 minutes. 5. Stir periodically; the sauce is ready once it's thickened slightly. Add the pork chops back into the pan, cover them with the sauce, and cook for 2 minutes. Serve.

Per Serving
Calories: 302 | Protein: 22g | Total Carbohydrates: 19g | Sugars: 17g | Fiber: 1g | Total Fat: 16g | Saturated Fat: 4g | Cholesterol: 55mg | Sodium: 753mg

Wine-Braised Short Ribs with Potatoes

Prep time: 20 minutes | Cook time: 1 hour 20 minutes | Serves 4

2 pounds (907g) bone-in English-style beef short ribs, trimmed
1 tablespoon extra-virgin olive oil
6 garlic cloves, minced
1 tablespoon minced fresh oregano or 1 teaspoon dried
½ cup dry red wine
2 tablespoons minced fresh parsley
¾ teaspoon table salt, divided
¼ teaspoon pepper
1 onion, chopped fine
2 tablespoons tomato paste
1 (14½ ounces / 411-g) can whole peeled tomatoes, drained with ¼ cup juice reserved, chopped coarse
1 pound (454 g) small red potatoes, unpeeled, halved

1. Pat short ribs dry with paper towels and sprinkle with ½ teaspoon salt and pepper. Using highest sauté function, heat oil in Instant Pot for 5 minutes (or until just smoking). Brown short ribs on all sides, 6 to 8 minutes; transfer to plate. 2. Add onion and remaining ¼ teaspoon salt to fat left in pot and cook, using highest sauté function, until onion is softened, about 3 minutes. Stir in garlic, tomato paste, and oregano and cook until fragrant, about 30 seconds. Stir in tomatoes and reserved juice and wine, scraping up any browned bits. Nestle short ribs meat side down into pot and add any accumulated juices. Lock lid in place and close pressure release valve. Select high pressure cook function and cook for 60 minutes. 3. Turn off Instant Pot and let pressure release naturally for 15 minutes. Quick-release any remaining pressure, then carefully remove lid, allowing steam to escape away from you. Transfer short ribs to serving dish, tent with aluminum foil, and let rest while preparing potatoes. 4. Strain braising liquid through fine-mesh strainer into fat separator; transfer solids to now-empty pot. Let braising liquid settle for 5 minutes, then pour 1½ cups defatted liquid and any accumulated juices into pot with solids; discard remaining liquid. Add potatoes. Lock lid in place and close pressure release valve. Select high pressure cook function and cook for 4 minutes. Turn off Instant Pot and quick-release pressure. Carefully remove lid, allowing steam to escape away from you. 5. Using slotted spoon, transfer potatoes to serving dish. Season sauce with salt and pepper to taste. Spoon sauce over short ribs and potatoes and sprinkle with parsley. Serve.

Per Serving
Cal: 340 | Total Fat: 13g | Sat Fat: 4.5g | Chol: 55mg | Sodium: 700mg | Total Carbs: 29g, Fiber: 3g, Total Sugar: 7g | Added Sugar: 0g | Protein: 21g

Greek Lamb Chops

Prep time: 10 minutes | Cook time: 6 to 8 hours | Serves 6

3 pounds (1.4 kg) lamb chops
Juice of 1 lemon
2 garlic cloves, minced
1 teaspoon sea salt
½ cup low-sodium beef broth
1 tablespoon extra-virgin olive oil
1 teaspoon dried oregano
½ teaspoon freshly ground black pepper

1. Put the lamb chops in a slow cooker. 2. In a small bowl, whisk together the beef broth, lemon juice, olive oil, garlic, oregano, salt, and pepper until blended. Pour the sauce over the lamb chops. 3. Cover the cooker and cook for 6 to 8 hours on Low heat.

Per Serving
Calories: 325 | Total fat: 13g | Sodium: 551mg | Carbohydrates: 1g | Fiber: 1g | Sugar: 1g | Protein: 47g

Beef and Goat Cheese Stuffed Peppers

Prep time: 10 minutes | Cook time: 30 minutes | Serves 4

1 pound (454 g) lean ground beef
2 Roma tomatoes, diced
½ yellow onion, diced
1 teaspoon salt
¼ teaspoon ground allspice
4 ounces (113 g) goat cheese
½ cup cooked brown rice
3 garlic cloves, minced
2 tablespoons fresh oregano, chopped
½ teaspoon black pepper
2 bell peppers, halved and seeded
¼ cup fresh parsley, chopped

1. Preheat the air fryer to 360°F (182°C). 2. In a large bowl, combine the ground beef, rice, tomatoes, garlic, onion, oregano, salt, pepper, and allspice. Mix well. 3. Divide the beef mixture equally into the halved bell peppers and top each with about 1 ounce (a quarter of the total) of the goat cheese. 4. Place the peppers into the air fryer basket in a single layer, making sure that they don't touch each other. Bake for 30 minutes. 5. Remove the peppers from the air fryer and top with fresh parsley before serving.

Per Serving
Calories: 298 | Total Fat: 12g | Saturated Fat: 7g | Protein: 32g | Total Carbohydrates: 17g | Fiber: 3g | Sugar: 2g | Cholesterol: 83mg

Greek Lamb Burgers

Prep time: 10 minutes | Cook time: 10 minutes | Serves 4

1 pound (454 g) ground lamb
4 tablespoons feta cheese, crumbled
½ teaspoon freshly ground black pepper
Buns, toppings, and tzatziki, for serving (optional)

1. Preheat a grill, grill pan, or lightly oiled skillet to high heat. 2. In a large bowl, using your hands, combine the lamb with the salt and pepper. 3. Divide the meat into 4 portions. Divide each portion in half to make a top and a bottom. Flatten each half into a 3-inch circle. Make a dent in the center of one of the halves and place 1 tablespoon of the feta cheese in the center. Place the second half of the patty on top of the feta cheese and press down to close the 2 halves together, making it resemble a round burger. 4. Cook the stuffed patty for 3 minutes on each side, for medium-well. Serve on a bun with your favorite toppings and tzatziki sauce, if desired.

Per Serving
Calories: 345 | Protein: 20g | Total Carbohydrates: 1g | Sugars: 0g | Fiber: 0g | Total Fat: 29g | Saturated Fat: 13g | Cholesterol: 91mg | Sodium: 462mg

Balsamic Pork Chops with Figs and Pears

Prep time: 15 minutes | Cook time: 13 minutes | Serves 2

- 2 (8 ounces / 227 g)) bone-in pork chops
- 1 teaspoon ground black pepper
- ¼ cup low-sodium chicken broth
- 2 tablespoons olive oil
- 3 medium pears, peeled, cored, and chopped
- ½ teaspoon salt
- ¼ cup balsamic vinegar
- 1 tablespoon dried mint
- 1 medium sweet onion, peeled and sliced
- 5 dried figs, stems removed and halved

1. Pat pork chops dry with a paper towel and season both sides with salt and pepper. Set aside. 2. In a small bowl, whisk together vinegar, broth, and mint. Set aside. 3. Press the Sauté button on the Instant Pot® and heat oil. Brown pork chops for 5 minutes per side. Remove chops and set aside. 4. Add vinegar mixture and scrape any brown bits from sides and bottom of pot. Layer onion slices in the pot, then scatter pears and figs over slices. Place pork chops on top. Press the Cancel button. 5. Close lid, set steam release to Sealing, press the Steam button, and set time to 3 minutes. When the timer beeps, let pressure release naturally for 10 minutes. Quick-release any remaining pressure until the float valve drops and then open lid. 6. Using a slotted spoon, transfer pork, onion, figs, and pears to a serving platter. Serve warm.

Per Serving
Calories: 672 | Fat: 32g | Protein: 27g | Sodium: 773mg | Fiber: 13 | Carbohydrates: 68g | Sugar: 36g

Lamb Kofta

Prep time: 15 minutes | Cook time: 10 minutes | Serves 4

- 1 pound (454 g) ground lamb
- 1½ teaspoons minced garlic (from 3 cloves), divided
- 1 teaspoon ground cumin
- 1–2 tablespoons olive oil
- 2 tablespoons tahini
- 1 tablespoon chopped fresh mint
- 2 teaspoons ground coriander
- 1 teaspoon kosher salt
- 2 tablespoons low-fat plain Greek yogurt
- 2 tablespoons fresh lemon juice

1. Coat a grill rack or grill pan with olive oil and prepare the grill to medium heat. 2. In a medium bowl, combine the lamb, mint, 1 teaspoon of the garlic, the coriander, cumin, and salt and mix until well blended. Divide into 8 balls and roll each ball into an elongated oval shape (like a football). Thread the meat onto metal skewers, 2 pieces per skewer, and brush with the oil. 3. Grill the skewers until cooked through and a thermometer inserted in the thickest part registers 160°F (71°C), turning once, 3 to 4 minutes per side. 4. In a small bowl, stir together the yogurt, tahini, lemon juice, and the remaining ½ teaspoon garlic. Serve the kofta with the sauce.

Per Serving
calories:278 | protein: 21g | carbohydrate: 4g | sugars: 1g | total fat: 20g | saturated fat: 7g | fiber: 1g | sodium: 549 mg

Pork Casserole with Fennel and Potatoes

Prep time: 20 minutes | Cook time: 6 to 8 hours | Serves 6

- 2 large fennel bulbs
- 2 pounds (907g) red potatoes, quartered
- 4 garlic cloves, minced
- 1 teaspoon dried parsley
- Freshly ground black pepper
- 3 pounds (1.4 kg) pork tenderloin, cut into 1½-inch pieces
- 1 cup low-sodium chicken broth
- 1½ teaspoons dried thyme
- 1 teaspoon sea salt
- ⅓ cup shredded Parmesan cheese

1. Cut the stalks off the fennel bulbs. Trim a little piece from the bottom of the bulbs to make them stable, then cut straight down through the bulbs to halve them. Cut the halves into quarters. Peel off and discard any wilted outer layers. Cut the fennel pieces crosswise into slices. 2. In a slow cooker, combine the fennel, pork, and potatoes. Stir to mix well. 3. In a small bowl, whisk together the chicken broth, garlic, thyme, parsley, and salt until combined. Season with pepper and whisk again. Pour the sauce over the pork. 4. Cover the cooker and cook for 6 to 8 hours on Low heat. 5. Top with Parmesan cheese for serving.

Per Serving
Calories: 918 | Total fat: 30g | Sodium: 1,001mg | Carbohydrates: 46g | Fiber: 8g | Sugar: 4g | Protein: 109g

Pork Tenderloin with Vegetable Ragu

Prep time: 25 minutes | Cook time: 18 minutes | Serves 6

- 2 tablespoons light olive oil, divided
- ¼ teaspoon salt
- 1 medium zucchini, trimmed and sliced
- 1 medium onion, peeled and chopped
- 1 (14½ ounces / 411-g) can diced tomatoes, drained
- ¼ teaspoon crushed red pepper flakes
- 1 tablespoon chopped fresh oregano
- ½ cup red wine
- 1 (1½-pound) pork tenderloin
- ¼ teaspoon ground black pepper
- 1 medium yellow squash, sliced
- 1 medium carrot, peeled and grated
- 2 cloves garlic, peeled and minced
- 1 tablespoon chopped fresh basil
- 1 sprig fresh thyme

1. Press the Sauté button on the Instant Pot® and heat 1 tablespoon oil. Season pork with salt and black pepper. Brown pork lightly on all sides, about 2 minutes per side. Transfer pork to a plate and set aside. 2. Add remaining 1 tablespoon oil to the pot. Add zucchini and squash, and cook until tender, about 5 minutes. Add onion and carrot, and cook until just softened, about 5 minutes. Add tomatoes, garlic, crushed red pepper flakes, basil, oregano, thyme, and red wine to pot, and stir well. Press the Cancel button. 3. Top vegetable mixture with browned pork. Close lid, set steam release to Sealing, press the Manual button, and set time to 3 minutes. When the timer beeps, quick-release the pressure until the float valve drops and open lid. Transfer pork to a cutting board and cut into 1" slices. Pour sauce on a serving platter and arrange pork slices on top. Serve immediately.

Per Serving
Calories: 190 | Fat: 7g | Protein: 23g | Sodium: 606mg | Fiber: 2g | Carbohydrates: 9g | Sugar: 3g

Hearty Stewed Beef in Tomato Sauce

Prep time: 20 minutes | Cook time: 1 hour 45 minutes | Serves 5

- 3 tablespoons extra virgin olive oil
- 1 medium onion (any variety), diced
- 4 garlic cloves, minced
- 2 tablespoons tomato paste
- 4 cloves
- 1 bay leaf
- 15 ounces (425g) canned crushed tomatoes or chopped fresh tomatoes
- 2 pounds (907g) boneless beef chuck, cut into 2-inch (5cm) chunks
- ⅓ cup white wine
- 1 cinnamon stick
- 4 allspice berries
- ¼ teaspoons freshly ground black pepper
- 1 cup hot water
- ½ teaspoons fine sea salt

1. Add the olive oil to a deep pan over medium heat. When the oil starts to shimmer, place half the beef in the pan. Brown the meat until a crust develops, about 3–4 minutes per side, then transfer the meat to a plate, and set aside. Repeat with the remaining pieces. 2. Add the onions to the pan and sauté for 3 minutes or until soft, using a wooden spatula to scrape the browned bits from the bottom of the pan. Add the garlic and sauté for 1 minute, then add the wine and deglaze the pan for 1 more minute, again using the wooden spatula to scrape any browned bits from the bottom of the pan. 3. Add the tomato paste to the pan while stirring rapidly, then add the cinnamon stick, cloves, allspice berries, bay leaf, black pepper, crushed tomatoes, and hot water. Mix well. 4. Add the beef back to the pan. Stir, then cover and reduce the heat to low. Simmer for 1 hour 30 minutes or until the beef is cooked through and tender, and the sauce has thickened. (If the sauce becomes too dry, add more hot water as needed.) 5. About 10 minutes before the cooking time is complete, add the sea salt and stir. When ready to serve, remove the cinnamon stick, bay leaf, allspice berries, and cloves. Store in the refrigerator for up to 3 days.

Per Serving
Calories: 565 | Total fat: 44g | Saturated fat: 15g | Carbohydrate: 10g | Protein: 33g

Giouvarlakia Soup

Prep time: 10 minutes | Cook time: 5 minutes | Serves 6

1 pound (454 g) lean ground beef	1 medium onion, peeled and grated
3 large eggs, divided	⅓ cup plus ½ cup Arborio rice, divided
1 teaspoon ground allspice	⅛ teaspoon ground nutmeg
¾ teaspoon salt, divided	¾ teaspoon ground black pepper, divided
8 cups low-sodium chicken broth	1 tablespoon all-purpose flour
2 tablespoons water	3 tablespoons lemon juice

1. In a large bowl, combine beef, onion, 1 egg, ⅓ cup rice, allspice, nutmeg, ¼ teaspoon salt, and ¼ teaspoon pepper. Roll the mixture into 1" balls. Set aside. 2. Add broth, meatballs, remaining ½ cup rice, and remaining ½ teaspoon each salt and pepper to the Instant Pot®. Close lid, set steam release to Sealing, press the Manual button, and set time to 5 minutes. When the timer beeps, let pressure release naturally for 10 minutes. Quick-release any remaining pressure until the float valve drops. Press the Cancel button and open lid. 3. In a large bowl, whisk together flour and water to form a slurry. Whisk in lemon juice and remaining 2 eggs. Continuing to whisk vigorously, slowly add a ladle of soup liquid into egg mixture. Continue whisking and slowly add another 3–4 ladles of soup (one at a time) into egg mixture. 4. Slowly stir egg mixture back into the soup. 5 Allow the soup to cool for 5 minutes and then serve it immediately.

Per Serving
Calories: 262 | Fat: 5g | Protein: 25g | Sodium: 670mg | Fiber: 0 | Carbohydrates: 18g | Sugar: 5g

Beef Meatballs in Garlic Cream Sauce

Prep time: 15 minutes | Cook time: 6 to 8 hours | Serves 4

For the sauce

1 cup low-sodium vegetable broth or low-sodium chicken broth	1 tablespoon extra-virgin olive oil
	2 garlic cloves, minced
1 tablespoon dried onion flakes	1 teaspoon dried rosemary
2 tablespoons freshly squeezed lemon juice	Pinch sea salt
Pinch freshly ground black pepper	

For the meatballs

1 pound (454 g) raw ground beef	1 large egg
2 tablespoons bread crumbs	1 teaspoon ground cumin
1 teaspoon salt	½ teaspoon freshly ground black pepper
To finish	2 cups plain Greek yogurt
2 tablespoons chopped fresh parsley	

To make the sauce:
In a medium bowl, whisk together the vegetable broth, olive oil, garlic, onion flakes, rosemary, lemon juice, salt, and pepper until combined.

To make the meatballs:
1. In a large bowl, mix together the ground beef, egg, bread crumbs, cumin, salt, and pepper until combined. Shape the meat mixture into 10 to 12 (2½-inch) meatballs. 2. Pour the sauce into the slow cooker. 3. Add the meatballs to the slow cooker. 4. Cover the cooker and cook for 6 to 8 hours on Low heat. 4. Stir in the yogurt. Replace the cover on the cooker and cook for 15 to 30 minutes on Low heat, or until the sauce has thickened. 5. Garnish with fresh parsley for serving.

Per Serving
Calories: 345 | Total fat: 20g | Sodium: 842mg | Carbohydrates: 13g | Fiber: 1g | Sugar: 8g | Protein: 29g

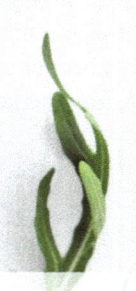

Chapter 4 Breakfasts

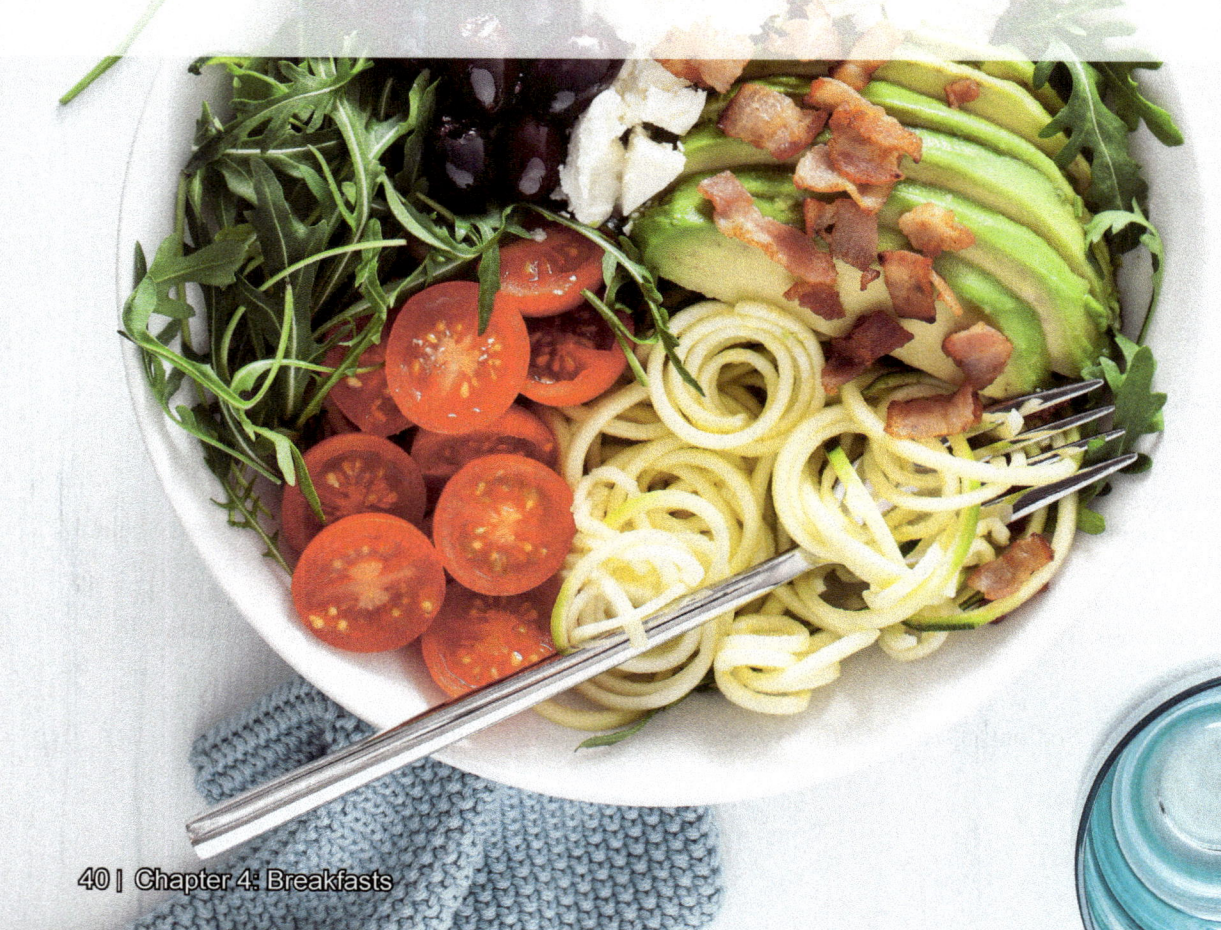

45 **Mediterranean Breakfast Pita Sandwiches** 42
46 **Fig and Ricotta Toast with Walnuts and Honey** 42
47 **Blueberry-Banana Bowl with Quinoa** 42
48 **Spinach Pie** 43
49 **Golden Egg Skillet** 43
50 **Greek Egg and Tomato Scramble** 44
51 **Avocado Toast with Smoked Trout** 44
52 **Garlicky Beans and Greens with Polenta** 44
53 **Strawberry Collagen Smoothie** 45
54 **Savory Cottage Cheese Breakfast Bowl** 45
55 **Greek Yogurt Parfait with Granola** 45
56 **Buckwheat Porridge with Fresh Fruit** 46
57 **Smoked Salmon Egg Scramble with Dill and Chives** 46
58 **Egg in a "Pepper Hole" with Avocado** 46
59 **Spinach and Feta Frittata** 47
60 **Spanish Tortilla with Potatoes and Peppers** 47
61 **Savory Parmesan Oatmeal** 48
62 **Egg and Pepper Pita** 48
63 **Whole Wheat Banana-Walnut Bread** 49
64 **Egg Salad with Red Pepper and Dill** 49

Mediterranean Breakfast Pita Sandwiches

Prep time: 5 minutes | Cook time: 7 minutes | Serves 2

2 eggs
¼ teaspoons fresh lemon juice
¼ teaspoons freshly ground black pepper
12 ¼-inch (.5cm) thick cucumber slices
2 tablespoons crumbled feta
½ teaspoons extra virgin olive oil

1 small avocado, peeled, halved, and pitted
Pinch of salt
8-inch (20cm) whole-wheat pocket pita bread, halved
6 oil-packed sun-dried tomatoes, rinsed, patted dry, and cut in half

1. Fill a small saucepan with water and place it over medium heat. When the water is boiling, use a slotted spoon to carefully lower the eggs into the water. Gently boil for 7 minutes, then remove the pan from the heat and transfer the eggs to a bowl of cold water. Set aside. 2. In a small bowl, mash the avocado with a fork and then add the lemon juice and salt. Mash to combine. 3. Peel and slice the eggs, then sprinkle the black pepper over the egg slices. 4. Spread half of the avocado mixture over one side of the pita half. Top the pita half with 1 sliced egg, 6 cucumber slices, and 6 sun-dried tomato pieces. 5. Sprinkle 1 tablespoon crumbled feta over the top and drizzle ¼ teaspoon olive oil over the feta. Repeat with the other pita half. Serve promptly.

Per Serving
Calories: 386 | Total fat: 20g | Saturated fat: 5g | Carbohydrate: 38g | Protein: 14g

Fig and Ricotta Toast with Walnuts and Honey

Prep time: 5 minutes | Cook time: 0 minutes | Serves 2

¼ cup ricotta cheese
4 figs, halved
1 teaspoon honey

2 pieces whole-wheat bread, toasted
2 tablespoons walnuts, chopped

1. Spread 2 tablespoons of ricotta cheese on each piece of toast. Add 4 fig halves to each piece of toast, pressing firmly to keep the figs in the ricotta. 2. Sprinkle 1 tablespoon of walnuts and drizzle ½ teaspoon of honey on each piece of toast.

Per Serving
Calories: 215 | Fat:10g | Protein: 7g | Carbs: 26g | Sugars: 9g | Fiber:3g | Sodium: 125mg | Cholesterol: 16mg

Blueberry-Banana Bowl with Quinoa

Prep time: 5 minutes | Cook time: 20 minutes | Serves 4

1½ cups water
2 tablespoons honey, divided
2 bananas (preferably frozen), sliced
½ cup dried cranberries
1 cup milk or nondairy milk of your choice

¾ cup uncooked quinoa, rinsed
1 cup blueberries (preferably frozen)
½ cup sliced almonds or crushed walnuts
1 cup granola

1. Combine the water and quinoa in a medium saucepan. Bring to a boil over medium-high heat, cover, reduce the heat to low, and simmer for 15 to 20 minutes, until the water has been absorbed. Remove from the heat and fluff the quinoa with a fork. 2. Evenly divide the quinoa among four bowls, about ½ cup for each bowl. Evenly divide the honey among the bowls and mix it in well. Top evenly with the blueberries, bananas, almonds, cranberries, granola, and milk. Serve.

Per Serving
Calories: 469 | Total fat: 15g | Total carbs: 77g | Sugar: 33g | Protein: 12g | Fiber: 9g | Sodium: 31mg

Spinach Pie

Prep time: 10 minutes | Cook time: 25 minutes | Serves 8

- Nonstick cooking spray
- 1 onion, chopped
- ¼ teaspoon garlic salt
- ¼ teaspoon ground nutmeg
- 1 cup grated Parmesan cheese, divided
- 4 hard-boiled eggs, halved
- 2 tablespoons extra-virgin olive oil
- 1 pound (454 g) frozen spinach, thawed
- ¼ teaspoon freshly ground black pepper
- 4 large eggs, divided
- 2 puff pastry doughs, (organic, if available), at room temperature

1. Preheat the oven to 350°F (177°C). Spray a baking sheet with nonstick cooking spray and set aside. 2. Heat a large sauté pan or skillet over medium-high heat. Put in the oil and onion and cook for about 5 minutes, until translucent. 3. Squeeze the excess water from the spinach, then add to the pan and cook, uncovered, so that any excess water from the spinach can evaporate. Add the garlic salt, pepper, and nutmeg. Remove from heat and set aside to cool. 4. In a small bowl, crack 3 eggs and mix well. Add the eggs and ½ cup Parmesan cheese to the cooled spinach mix. 5. On the prepared baking sheet, roll out the pastry dough. Layer the spinach mix on top of dough, leaving 2 inches around each edge. 6. Once the spinach is spread onto the pastry dough, place hard-boiled egg halves evenly throughout the pie, then cover with the second pastry dough. Pinch the edges closed. 7. Crack the remaining egg in a small bowl and mix well. Brush the egg wash over the pastry dough. 8. Bake for 15 to 20 minutes, until golden brown and warmed through.

Per Serving

Calories: 417 | Protein: 17g | Total Carbohydrates: 25g | Sugars: 1g | Fiber: 3g | Total Fat: 28g | Saturated Fat: 7g | Cholesterol: 210mg | Sodium: 490mg

Golden Egg Skillet

Prep time: 15 minutes | Cook time: 20 minutes | Serves 2

- 2 tablespoons extra-virgin avocado oil or ghee
- 1 clove garlic, minced
- 3½ ounces (100 g) Swiss chard or collard greens, stalks and leaves separated, chopped
- 1 teaspoon Dijon or yellow mustard
- ¼ teaspoon black pepper
- 4 large eggs
- 2 tablespoons extra-virgin olive oil
- 2 medium (30 g/1.1 ounces) spring onions, white and green parts separated, sliced
- 1 medium (200 g/7 ounces) zucchini, sliced into coins
- 2 tablespoons water
- ½ teaspoon ground turmeric
- Salt, to taste
- ¾ cup (85 g/3 ounces) grated Manchego or Pecorino Romano cheese

1. Preheat the oven to 360°F (182°C) fan assisted or 400°F (204°C) conventional. 2. Grease a large, ovenproof skillet (with a lid) with the avocado oil. Cook the white parts of the spring onions and the garlic for about 1 minute, until just fragrant. Add the chard stalks, zucchini, and water. Stir, then cover with a lid. Cook over medium-low heat for about 10 minutes or until the zucchini is tender. Add the mustard, turmeric, pepper, and salt. Add the chard leaves and cook until just wilted. 3. Use a spatula to make 4 wells in the mixture. Crack an egg into each well and cook until the egg whites start to set while the yolks are still runny. Top with the cheese, transfer to the oven, and bake for 5 to 7 minutes. Remove from the oven and sprinkle with the reserved spring onions. Drizzle with the olive oil and serve warm.

Per Serving

Total carbs: 8.1g | Fiber: 2.5g | Net Carbs: 5.6g | Protein: 25.9g | Fat: 48.2g (of which saturated: 14.4g) | Calories: 560

Greek Egg and Tomato Scramble

Prep time: 10 minutes | Cook time: 25 minutes | Serves 4

¼ cup extra-virgin olive oil, divided
¼ cup finely minced red onion
½ teaspoon dried oregano or 1 to 2 teaspoons chopped fresh oregano
8 large eggs
¼ teaspoon freshly ground black pepper
¼ cup chopped fresh mint leaves
1½ cups chopped fresh tomatoes
2 garlic cloves, minced
½ teaspoon dried thyme or 1 to 2 teaspoons chopped fresh thyme
½ teaspoon salt
¾ cup crumbled feta cheese

1. In large skillet, heat the olive oil over medium heat. Add the chopped tomatoes and red onion and sauté until tomatoes are cooked through and soft, 10 to 12 minutes. 2. Add the garlic, oregano, and thyme and sauté another 2 to 4 minutes, until fragrant and liquid has reduced. 3. In a medium bowl, whisk together the eggs, salt, and pepper until well combined. 4. Add the eggs to the skillet, reduce the heat to low, and scramble until set and creamy, using a spatula to move them constantly, 3 to 4 minutes. Remove the skillet from the heat, stir in the feta and mint, and serve warm.

Per Serving
Calories: 338 | Total Fat: 28g | Total Carbs: 6g | Net Carbs: 5g | Fiber: 1g | Protein: 16g | Sodium: 570mg

Avocado Toast with Smoked Trout

Prep time: 10 minutes | Cook time: 0 minutes | Serves 2

1 avocado, peeled and pitted
¾ teaspoon ground cumin
¼ teaspoon red pepper flakes, plus more for sprinkling
2 pieces whole-wheat bread, toasted
2 teaspoons lemon juice, plus more for serving
¼ teaspoon kosher salt
¼ teaspoon lemon zest
1 (3.75 ounces / 106-g) can smoked trout

1. In a medium bowl, mash together the avocado, lemon juice, cumin, salt, red pepper flakes, and lemon zest. 2. Spread half the avocado mixture on each piece of toast. Top each piece of toast with half the smoked trout. Garnish with a pinch of red pepper flakes (if desired), and/or a sprinkle of lemon juice (if desired).

Per Serving
Calories: 300 | Fat: 20g | Protein: 11g | Carbs: 21g | Sugars: 1g | Fiber: 6g | Sodium: 390mg | Cholesterol: 23mg

Garlicky Beans and Greens with Polenta

Prep time: 5 minutes | Cook time: 20 minutes | Serves 4

2 tablespoons olive oil, divided
4 cloves garlic, minced
4 cups chopped greens, such as kale, mustard greens, collards, or chard
Kosher salt and ground black pepper, to taste
1 roll (18 ounces / 510 g) precooked polenta, cut into ½"-thick slices
2 tomatoes, seeded and diced
1 can (15 ounces / 425-g) small white beans, drained and rinsed

1. In a large skillet over medium heat, warm 1 tablespoon of the oil. Cook the polenta slices, flipping once, until golden and crispy, about 5 minutes per side. Remove the polenta and keep warm. 2. Add the remaining 1 tablespoon oil to the skillet. Cook the garlic until softened, 1 minute. Add the greens, tomatoes, and beans and cook until the greens are wilted and bright green and the beans are heated through, 10 minutes. Season to taste with the salt and pepper. To serve, top the polenta with the beans and greens.

Per Serving
calories: 376 | protein: 16g | carbohydrates: 36g | sugars: 4g | total fat: 20g | saturated fat: 5g | fiber: 4g | sodium: 678mg

Strawberry Collagen Smoothie

Prep time: 5 minutes | Cook time: 0 minutes | Serves 1

3 ounces (85 g) fresh or frozen strawberries
¼ cup (60 ml) coconut cream or goat's cream
1 tablespoon (8 g/0.3 ounces) chia seeds or flax meal
¼ teaspoon vanilla powder or 1 teaspoon unsweetened vanilla extract
Optional: ice cubes, to taste

¾ cup (180 ml) unsweetened almond milk
1 large egg
2 tablespoons (14 g/0.5 ounces) grass-fed collagen powder
Zest from ½ lemon
1 tablespoon (15 ml) macadamia oil

1. Place all of the ingredients in a blender and pulse until smooth and frothy. Serve immediately.

Per Serving
Total carbs: 15.6 g | Fiber: 6.4 g | Net Carbs: 9.2 g | Protein: 23.5 g | Fat: 43.6 g (of which saturated: 22.6 g) | Calories: 519 kcal

Savory Cottage Cheese Breakfast Bowl

Prep time: 10 minutes | Cook time: 0 minutes | Serves 4

2 cups low-fat cottage cheese
½ teaspoon ground black pepper
1 large tomato, chopped
¼ cup pitted kalamata olives, halved

2 tablespoons chopped mixed fresh herbs, such as basil, dill, flat-leaf parsley, and oregano
1 small cucumber, peeled and chopped
1 tablespoon extra-virgin olive oil

1. In a medium bowl, combine the cottage cheese, herbs, and pepper. Add the tomato, cucumber, and olives and gently stir to combine. Drizzle with the oil to serve.

Per Serving
Calories: 181 | Protein: 15g | Carbohydrates: 8g | Sugars: 5g | Total Fat: 10g | Saturated Fat: 2g | Fiber: 1g | Sodium: 788mg

Greek Yogurt Parfait with Granola

Prep time: 10 minutes | Cook time: 30 minutes | Serves 4

For the Granola:
¼ cup honey or maple syrup
2 teaspoons vanilla extract
3 cups gluten-free rolled oats
¼ cup sunflower seeds
For the Parfait:
2 cups plain Greek yogurt

2 tablespoons vegetable oil
½ teaspoon kosher salt
1 cup mixed raw and unsalted nuts, chopped
1 cup unsweetened dried cherries

1 cup fresh fruit, chopped (optional)

To Make the Granola:
1. Preheat the oven to 325°F (163°C). Line a baking sheet with parchment paper or foil. 2. Heat the honey, oil, vanilla, and salt in a small saucepan over medium heat. Simmer for 2 minutes and stir together well. 3. In a large bowl, combine the oats, nuts, and seeds. Pour the warm oil mixture over the top and toss well. Spread in a single layer on the prepared baking sheet. Bake for 30 minutes, stirring halfway through. Remove from the oven and add in the dried cherries. Cool completely and store in an airtight container at room temperature for up to 3 months. To Make the Parfait: For one serving: In a bowl or lowball drinking glass, spoon in ½ cup yogurt, ½ cup granola, and ¼ cup fruit (if desired). Layer in whatever pattern you like.

Per Serving
Calories: 370 | Fat: 144g | Protein: 19g | Carbs: 44g | Sugars: 21g | Fiber: 6g | Sodium: 100mg | Cholesterol: 6mg

Buckwheat Porridge with Fresh Fruit

Prep time: 10 minutes | Cook time: 6 minutes | Serves 4

1 cup buckwheat groats, rinsed and drained
½ cup chopped pitted dates
¼ teaspoon ground cinnamon
½ teaspoon vanilla extract
1 cup raspberries
2 tablespoons balsamic vinegar

3 cups water
1 tablespoon light olive oil
¼ teaspoon salt
1 cup blueberries
1 cup hulled and quartered strawberries

1. Place buckwheat, water, dates, oil, cinnamon, and salt in the Instant Pot® and stir well. Close lid and set steam release to Sealing. Press the Manual button and set time to 6 minutes. 2. When the timer beeps, let pressure release naturally, about 20 minutes. Open lid and stir in vanilla. 3. While buckwheat cooks, combine blueberries, raspberries, strawberries, and vinegar in a medium bowl. Stir well. Top porridge with berry mixture. Serve hot.

Per Serving
Calories: 318 | Fat: 5g | Protein: 6g | Sodium: 151mg | Fiber: 9g | Carbohydrates: 64g | Sugar: 21g

Smoked Salmon Egg Scramble with Dill and Chives

Prep time: 5 minutes | Cook time: 5 minutes | Serves 2

4 large eggs
1 tablespoon fresh chives, minced
¼ teaspoon kosher salt
2 teaspoons extra-virgin olive oil

1 tablespoon milk
1 tablespoon fresh dill, minced
⅛ teaspoon freshly ground black pepper
2 ounces (57 g) smoked salmon, thinly sliced

1. In a large bowl, whisk together the eggs, milk, chives, dill, salt, and pepper. 2. Heat the olive oil in a medium skillet or sauté pan over medium heat. Add the egg mixture and cook for about 3 minutes, stirring occasionally. 3. Add the salmon and cook until the eggs are set but moist, about 1 minute.

Per Serving
Calories: 325 | Fat: 26g | Protein: 23g | Carbs: 1g | Sugars: 1g | Fiber: 0g | Sodium: 455mg | Cholesterol: 399mg

Egg in a "Pepper Hole" with Avocado

Prep time: 15 minutes | Cook time: 5 minutes | Serves 4

4 bell peppers, any color
8 large eggs
¼ teaspoon freshly ground black pepper, divided
¼ cup red onion, diced
Juice of ½ lime

1 tablespoon extra-virgin olive oil
¾ teaspoon kosher salt, divided
1 avocado, peeled, pitted, and diced
¼ cup fresh basil, chopped

1. Stem and seed the bell peppers. Cut 2 (2-inch-thick) rings from each pepper. Chop the remaining bell pepper into small dice, and set aside. 2. Heat the olive oil in a large skillet over medium heat. Add 4 bell pepper rings, then crack 1 egg in the middle of each ring. Season with ¼ teaspoon of the salt and ⅛ teaspoon of the black pepper. Cook until the egg whites are mostly set but the yolks are still runny, 2 to 3 minutes. Gently flip and cook 1 additional minute for over easy. Move the egg-bell pepper rings to a platter or onto plates, and repeat with the remaining 4 bell pepper rings. 3. In a medium bowl, combine the avocado, onion, basil, lime juice, reserved diced bell pepper, the remaining ¼ teaspoon kosher salt, and the remaining ⅛ teaspoon black pepper. Divide among the 4 plates.

Per Serving
Calories: 270 | Fat: 19g | Protein: 15g | Carbs: 12g | Sugars: 6g | Fiber: 5g | Sodium: 360mg | Cholesterol: 370mg

Spinach and Feta Frittata

Prep time: 10 minutes | Cook time: 26 minutes | Serves 4

1 tablespoon olive oil	½ medium onion, peeled and chopped
½ medium red bell pepper, seeded and chopped	2 cups chopped fresh baby spinach
1 cup water	1 cup crumbled feta cheese
6 large eggs, beaten	¼ cup low-fat plain Greek yogurt
½ teaspoon salt	½ teaspoon ground black pepper

1. Press the Sauté button on the Instant Pot® and heat oil. Add onion and bell pepper, and cook until tender, about 8 minutes. Add spinach and cook until wilted, about 3 minutes. Press the Cancel button and transfer vegetables to a medium bowl to cool. Wipe out inner pot. 2. Place the rack in the Instant Pot® and add water. Spray a 1.5-liter baking dish with nonstick cooking spray. Drain excess liquid from spinach mixture, then add to dish with cheese. 3. In a separate medium bowl, mix eggs, yogurt, salt, and black pepper until well combined. Pour over vegetable and cheese mixture. Cover dish tightly with foil, then gently lower into machine. 4. Close lid, set steam release to Sealing, press the Manual button, and set time to 15 minutes. When the timer beeps, let pressure release naturally for 10 minutes, then quick-release any remaining pressure until the float valve drops. Press the Cancel button and open lid. Let stand for 10–15 minutes before carefully removing dish from pot. 5. Run a thin knife around the edge of the frittata and turn it out onto a serving platter. Serve warm.

Per Serving

Calories: 303 | Fat: 23g | Protein: 21g | Sodium: 1,096mg | Fiber: 2 g | Carbohydrates: 7g | Sugar: 2g

Spanish Tortilla with Potatoes and Peppers

Prep time : 5 minutes | Cook time: 50 minutes | Serves 6

½ cup olive oil, plus 2 tablespoons, divided	2 pounds (907g) baking potatoes, peeled and cut into ¼-inch slices
2 onions, thinly sliced	
1 roasted red pepper, drained and cut into strips	6 eggs
2 teaspoons salt	1 teaspoon freshly ground black pepper

1. In a large skillet over medium heat, heat ½ cup of the olive oil. Add the potatoes and cook, stirring occasionally, until the potatoes are tender, about 20 minutes. Remove the potatoes from the pan with a slotted spoon and discard the remaining oil. 2. In a medium skillet over medium heat, heat the remaining 2 tablespoons of olive oil. Add the onions and cook, stirring frequently, until softened and golden brown, about 10 minutes. Remove the onions from the pan with a slotted spoon, leaving the oil in the pan, and add them to the potatoes. Add the pepper slices to the potatoes as well. 3. In a large bowl, whisk together the eggs, salt, and pepper. Add the cooked vegetables to the egg mixture and gently toss to combine. 4. Heat the medium skillet over low heat. Add the egg-vegetable mixture to the pan and cook for about 10 minutes, until the bottom is lightly browned. Use a spatula to loosen the tortilla and transfer the whole thing to a large plate, sliding it out of the pan so that the browned side is on the bottom. Invert the skillet over the tortilla and then lift the plate to flip it back into the skillet with the browned side on top. Return to the stove and continue to cook over low heat until the tortilla is fully set in the center, about 5 more minutes. 5. Serve the tortilla warm or at room temperature.

Per Serving:

Calories: 370 | Total Fat: 26g | Saturated Fat: 5g | Carbs: 29g | Protein: 9g | Sodium: 876mg | Fiber: 5g

Savory Parmesan Oatmeal

Prep timePrep Time: 10 minutes | Cook Time: 20 minutes | Serves 2

1 tablespoon olive oil
1 ounce (about 2 thin slices) prosciutto, minced
¾ cup gluten-free old-fashioned oats
1½ cups water, unsalted, or low-sodium chicken stock
Salt
¼ cup minced onion
2 cups greens (arugula, baby spinach, chopped kale, or Swiss chard)
2 tablespoons Parmesan cheese
Pinch freshly ground black pepper

1. Heat the olive oil in a saucepan over medium-high heat. Add the onion and prosciutto and sauté for 4 minutes, or until the prosciutto starts to crisp and the onion turns golden. 2. Add the greens and stir until they begin to wilt. Transfer this mixture to a bowl. 3. Add the oats to the pan and let them toast for about 2 minutes. Add the water or chicken stock and bring the oats to a boil. Reduce the heat to low, cover the pan, and let the oats cook for 10 minutes, or until the liquid is absorbed and the oats are tender. 4. Stir the Parmesan cheese into the oats, and add the onions, prosciutto, and greens back to the pan. Add additional water if needed, so the oats are creamy and not dry. 5. Stir well and add salt and freshly ground black pepper to taste.

Per Serving
Calories: 258 | Total fat: 12g | Total carbs: 29g | Fiber: 6g | Sugar: 1g | Protein: 11g | Sodium: 260mg | Cholesterol: 13mg

Egg and Pepper Pita

Prep time: 10 minutes | Cook time: 10 minutes | Serves 4

2 pita breads
1 red or yellow bell pepper, diced
4 large eggs, beaten
Freshly ground black pepper
2 avocados, sliced
2 tablespoons chopped scallion, green part only, for garnish
2 tablespoons olive oil
2 zucchini, quartered lengthwise and sliced
Sea salt
Pinch dried oregano
½ to ¾ cup crumbled feta cheese
Hot sauce, for serving

1. In a large skillet, heat the pitas over medium heat until warmed through and lightly toasted, about 2 minutes. Remove the pitas from the skillet and set aside. 2. In the same skillet, heat the olive oil over medium heat. Add the bell pepper and zucchini and sauté for 4 to 5 minutes. Add the eggs and season with salt, black pepper, and the oregano. Cook, stirring, for 2 to 3 minutes, until the eggs are cooked through. Remove from the heat. 3. Slice the pitas in half crosswise and fill each half with the egg mixture. Divide the avocado and feta among the pita halves. Garnish with the scallion and serve with hot sauce.

Per Serving
Calories: 476 | Total fat: 31g | Total carbs: 36g | Sugar: 8g | Protein: 17g | Fiber: 11g | Sodium: 455mg

Whole Wheat Banana-Walnut Bread

Prep time: 10 minutes | Cook time: 23 minutes | Serves 6

Olive oil cooking spray
1 large egg
¼ cup olive oil
2 tablespoons raw honey
¼ teaspoon salt
½ teaspoon ground cinnamon

2 ripe medium bananas
¼ cup nonfat plain Greek yogurt
½ teaspoon vanilla extract
1 cup whole wheat flour
¼ teaspoon baking soda
¼ cup chopped walnuts

1. Preheat the air fryer to 360°F (182°C). Lightly coat the inside of a 8-by-4-inch loaf pan with olive oil cooking spray. (Or use two 5 ½-by-3-inch loaf pans.) 2. In a large bowl, mash the bananas with a fork. Add the egg, yogurt, olive oil, vanilla, and honey. Mix until well combined and mostly smooth. 3. Sift the whole wheat flour, salt, baking soda, and cinnamon into the wet mixture, then stir until just combined. Do not overmix. 4. Gently fold in the walnuts. 5. Pour into the prepared loaf pan and spread to distribute evenly. 6. Place the loaf pan in the air fryer basket and bake for 20 to 23 minutes, or until golden brown on top and a toothpick inserted into the center comes out clean. 7. Allow to cool for 5 minutes before serving.

Per Serving
Calories: 255 | Total Fat: 14g | Saturated Fat: 2g | Protein: 6g | Total Carbohydrates: 30g | Fiber: 4g | Sugar: 11g | Cholesterol: 31mg

Egg Salad with Red Pepper and Dill

Prep time: 5 minutes | Cook time: 10 minutes | Serves 6

6 large eggs
1 tablespoon olive oil
¼ teaspoon salt
½ cup low-fat plain Greek yogurt

1 cup water
1 medium red bell pepper, seeded and chopped
¼ teaspoon ground black pepper
2 tablespoons chopped fresh dill

1. Have ready a large bowl of ice water. Place rack or egg holder into bottom of the Instant Pot®. 2. Arrange eggs on rack or holder and add water to the Instant Pot®. Close lid, set steam release to Sealing, press the Manual button, and set time to 5 minutes. 3. When the timer beeps, let pressure release naturally for 5 minutes, then quick-release the remaining pressure until the float valve drops. Press the Cancel button and open lid. Carefully transfer eggs to the bowl of ice water. Let stand in ice water for 10 minutes, then peel, chop, and add eggs to a medium bowl. 4. Clean out pot, dry well, and return to machine. Press the Sauté button and heat oil. Add bell pepper, salt, and black pepper. Cook, stirring often, until bell pepper is tender, about 5 minutes. Transfer to bowl with eggs. 5. Add yogurt and dill to bowl, and fold to combine. Cover and chill for 1 hour before serving.

Per Serving
Calories: 111 | Fat: 8g | Protein: 8g | Sodium: 178mg | Fiber: 0g | Carbohydrates: 3g | Sugar: 1g

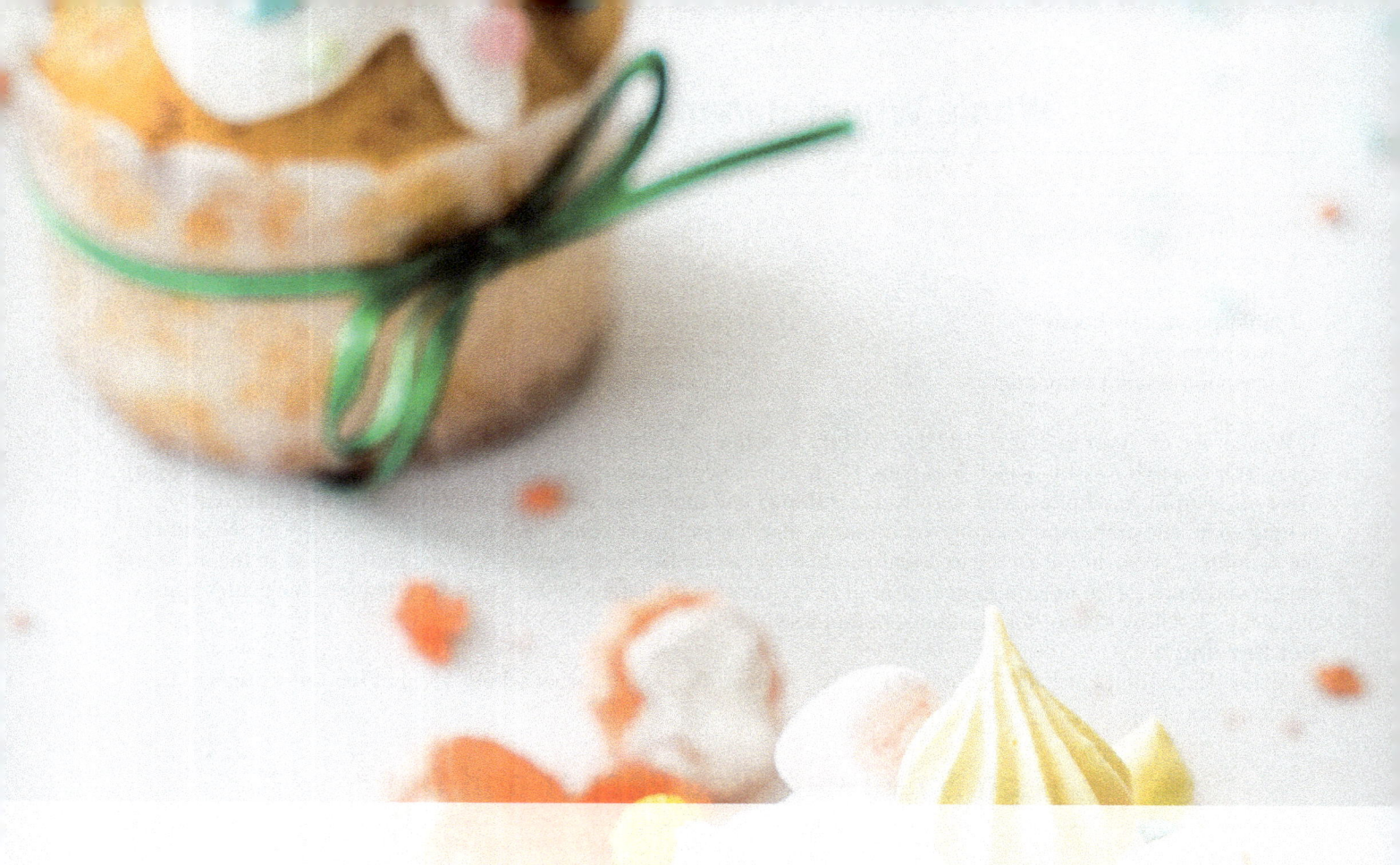

Chapter 5   Desserts

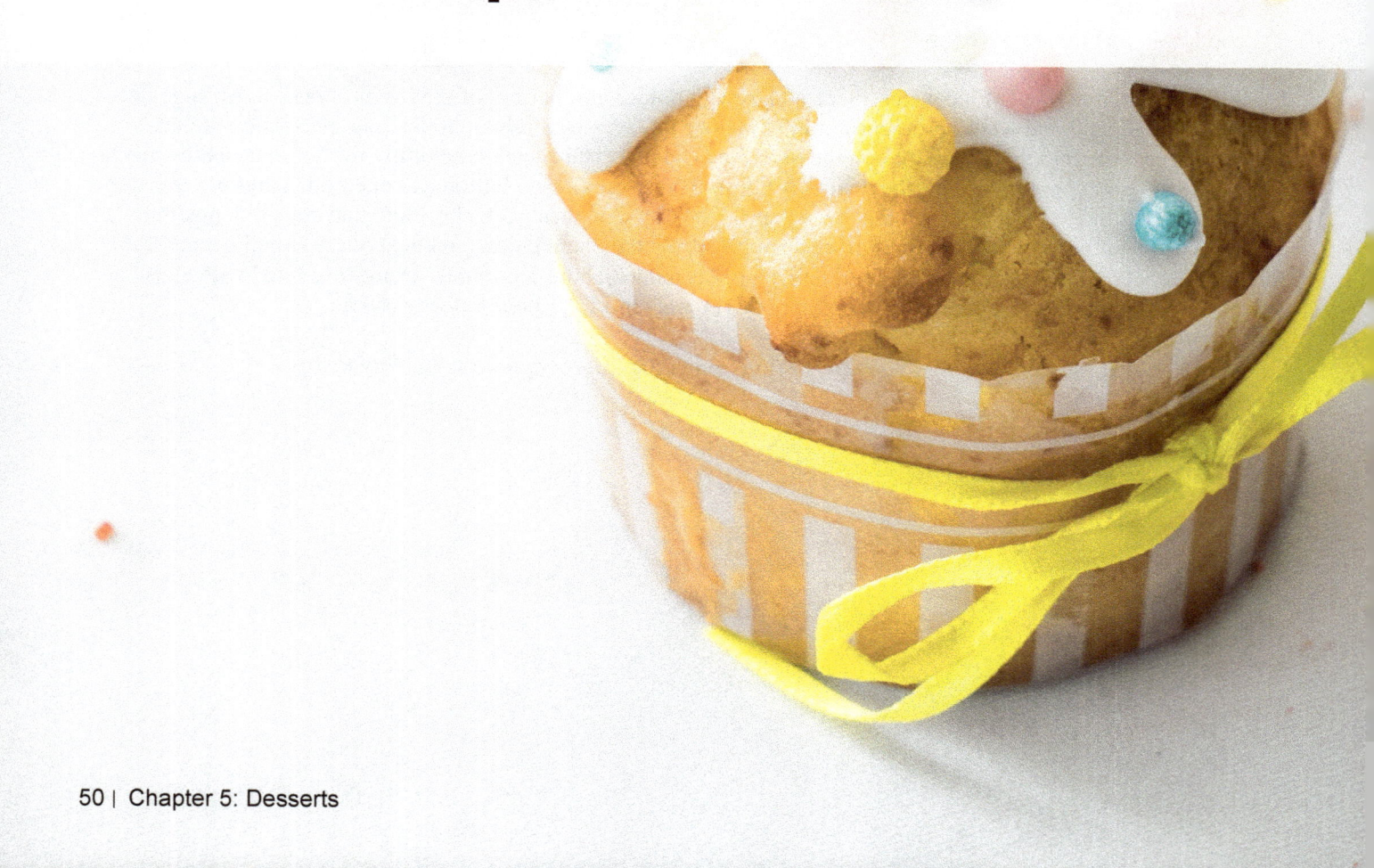

65 **Toasted Almonds with Honey** 52
66 **Poached Pears with Greek Yogurt and Pistachio** 52
67 **Pears Poached in Pomegranate and Wine** 52
68 **Lemon Coconut Cake** 53
69 **Crunchy Sesame Cookies** 53
70 **Light and Lemony Olive Oil Cupcakes** 54
71 **Dark Chocolate Bark with Fruit and Nuts** 54
72 **Greek Yogurt with Honey and Pomegranates** 54
73 **Individual Meringues with Strawberries, Mint, and Toasted Coconut** 55
74 **Crispy Apple Phyllo Tart** 55
75 **Red Wine–Poached Figs with Ricotta and Almond** 56
76 **Ricotta-Lemon Cheesecake** 56
77 **Creamy Rice Pudding** 56
78 **Fruit Compote** 57
79 **Lightened-Up Baklava Rolls** 57
80 **Cinnamon-Stewed Dried Plums with Greek Yogurt** 58
81 **Chocolate Hazelnut "Powerhouse" Truffles** 58
82 **Strawberry-Pomegranate Molasses Sauce** 59
83 **Greek Yogurt Ricotta Mousse** 59
84 **Blueberry Compote** 59
85 **Figs with Mascarpone and Honey** 60
86 **Spiced Baked Pears with Mascarpone** 60

Toasted Almonds with Honey

Prep time: 15 minutes | Cook time: 5 minutes | Serves 4

½ cup raw almonds

3 tablespoons good-quality honey, plus more if desired

1. Fill a medium saucepan three-quarters full with water and bring to a boil over high heat. Add the almonds and cook for 1 minute. Drain the almonds in a fine-mesh sieve and rinse them under cold water to cool and stop the cooking. Remove the skins from the almonds by rubbing them in a clean kitchen towel. Place the almonds on a paper towel to dry. 2. In the same saucepan, combine the almonds and honey and cook over medium heat until the almonds get a little golden, 4 to 5 minutes. Remove from the heat and let cool completely, about 15 minutes, before serving or storing.

Per Serving
Calories: 151 | Total fat: 9g | Total carbs: 17g | Sugar: 14g | Protein: 4g | Fiber: 2g | Sodium: 1mg

Poached Pears with Greek Yogurt and Pistachio

Prep time: 10 minutes | Cook time: 3 minutes | Serves 8

2 cups water
¼ cup lemon juice
1 teaspoon vanilla bean paste
1 cup low-fat plain Greek yogurt

1¾ cups apple cider
1 cinnamon stick
4 large Bartlett pears, peeled
½ cup unsalted roasted pistachio meats

1. Add water, apple cider, lemon juice, cinnamon, vanilla, and pears to the Instant Pot®. Close lid, set steam release to Sealing, press the Manual button, and set time to 3 minutes. 2. When the timer beeps, quick-release the pressure until the float valve drops. Press the Cancel button and open lid. With a slotted spoon remove pears to a plate and allow to cool to room temperature. 3. To serve, carefully slice pears in half with a sharp paring knife and scoop out core with a melon baller. Lay pear halves on dessert plates or in shallow bowls. Top with yogurt and garnish with pistachios. Serve immediately.

Per Serving
Calories: 181 | Fat: 7g | Protein: 7g | Sodium: 11mg | Fiber: 4g | Carbohydrates: 23g | Sugar: 15g

Pears Poached in Pomegranate and Wine

Prep time: 5 minutes | Cook time: 60 minutes | Serves 4

4 ripe, firm Bosc pears, peeled, left whole, and stems left intact
1½ cups pomegranate juice
1 cup sweet, white dessert wine, such as vin santo
½ cup pomegranate seeds (seeds from about ½ whole fruit)

1. Slice off a bit of the bottom of each pear to create a flat surface so that the pears can stand upright. If desired, use an apple corer to remove the cores of the fruit, working from the bottom. 2. Lay the pears in a large saucepan on their sides and pour the juice and wine over the top. Set over medium-high heat and bring to a simmer. Cover the pan, reduce the heat, and let the pears simmer, turning twice, for about 40 minutes, until the pears are tender. Transfer the pears to a shallow bowl, leaving the cooking liquid in the saucepan. 3. Turn the heat under the saucepan to high and bring the poaching liquid to a boil. Cook, stirring frequently, for about 15 to 20 minutes, until the liquid becomes thick and syrupy and is reduced to about ½ cup. 4. Spoon a bit of the syrup onto each of 4 serving plates and top each with a pear, sitting it upright. Drizzle a bit more of the sauce over the pears and garnish with the pomegranate seeds. Serve immediately.

Per Serving
Calories: 208 | Total Fat: 0g | Saturated Fat: 0g | Carbs: 46g | Protein: 1g | Sodium: 7mg | Fiber: 7g

Lemon Coconut Cake

Prep time: 5 minutes | Cook time: 40 minutes | Serves 9

BASE
6 large eggs, separated
1 tablespoon (15 ml) fresh lemon juice
2 cups (200 g/7 ounces) almond flour
¼ cup (25 g/0.9 ounces) collagen powder
1 teaspoon vanilla powder or 1 tablespoon (15 ml) unsweetened vanilla extract

⅓ cup (80 ml) melted ghee or virgin coconut oil
Zest of 2 lemons (12 g/0.4 ounces)
½ cup (60 g/2.1 ounces) coconut flour
1 teaspoon baking soda
Optional: low-carb sweetener, to taste

TOPPING
½ cup (30 g/1.1 ounces) unsweetened large coconut flakes
1 cup (240 ml) heavy whipping cream or coconut cream
¼ cup (60 g/2.1 ounces) mascarpone, more heavy whipping cream, or coconut cream
½ teaspoon vanilla powder or 1½ teaspoons unsweetened vanilla extract

1. Preheat the oven to 285°F (140°C) fan assisted or 320°F (160°C) conventional. Line a baking tray with parchment paper (or use a silicone tray). A square 8 × 8–inch (20 × 20 cm) or a rectangular tray of similar size will work best. 2. To make the base: Whisk the egg whites in a bowl until stiff peaks form. In a separate bowl, whisk the egg yolks, melted ghee, lemon juice, and lemon zest. In a third bowl, mix the almond flour, coconut flour, collagen, baking soda, vanilla and optional sweetener. 3. Add the whisked egg yolk–ghee mixture into the dry mixture and combine well. Gently fold in the egg whites, trying not to deflate them. 4. Pour into the baking tray. Bake for 35 to 40 minutes, until lightly golden on top and set inside. Remove from the oven and let cool completely before adding the topping. 5. To make the topping: Preheat the oven to 350°F (177°C) fan assisted or 380°F (193°C) conventional. Place the coconut flakes on a baking tray and bake for 2 to 3 minutes. Remove from the oven and set aside to cool. 6. Once the cake is cool, place the cream, mascarpone, and vanilla in a bowl. Whip until soft peaks form. Spread on top of the cooled cake and top with the toasted coconut flakes. 7. To store, refrigerate for up to 5 days or freeze for up to 3 months. Coconut flakes will soften in the fridge. If you want to keep them crunchy, sprinkle on top of each slice before serving.

Per Serving
Total carbs: 8.3 g | Fiber: 4.1 g | Net Carbs: 4.2 g | Protein: 13.6 g | Fat: 38.6 g (of which saturated: 17.8 g) | Calories: 432

Crunchy Sesame Cookies

Prep time: 10 minutes | Cook time: 15 minutes | Yield 14 to 16

1 cup sesame seeds, hulled
8 tablespoons (1 stick) salted butter, softened
1¼ cups flour

1 cup sugar
2 large eggs

1. Preheat the oven to 350°F (177°C). Toast the sesame seeds on a baking sheet for 3 minutes. Set aside and let cool. 2. Using a mixer, cream together the sugar and butter. 3. Add the eggs one at a time until well-blended. 4. Add the flour and toasted sesame seeds and mix until well-blended. 5. Drop spoonfuls of cookie dough onto a baking sheet and form them into round balls, about 1-inch in diameter, similar to a walnut. 6. Put in the oven and bake for 5 to 7 minutes or until golden brown. 7. Let the cookies cool and enjoy.

Per Serving
Calories: 218 | Protein: 4g | Total Carbohydrates: 25g | Sugars: 14g | Fiber: 2g | Total Fat: 12g | Saturated Fat: 5g | Cholesterol: 44mg | Sodium: 58mg

Light and Lemony Olive Oil Cupcakes

Prep time: 10 minutes | Cook time: 24 minutes | Serves 18

2 cups all-purpose flour
1 cup granulated sugar
2 eggs
1 teaspoon pure vanilla extract
Zest of 2 lemons
1 tablespoon lemon juice
4 teaspoons baking powder
1 cup extra virgin olive oil
7 ounces (200g) 2% Greek yogurt
4 tablespoons fresh lemon juice
For the glaze
5 tablespoons powdered sugar

1. Preheat the oven to 350°F (177°C). Line a 12-cup muffin pan with cupcake liners and then line a second pan with 6 liners. Set aside. 2. In a medium bowl, combine the flour and baking powder. Whisk and set aside. 3. In a large bowl, combine the sugar and olive oil, and mix until smooth. Add the eggs, one at a time, and mix well. Add the Greek yogurt, vanilla extract, lemon juice, and lemon zest. Mix until well combined. 4. Add the flour mixture to the batter, ½ cup at a time, while continuously mixing. 5. Spoon the batter into the liners, filling each liner two-thirds full. Bake for 22–25 minutes or until a toothpick inserted into the center of a cupcake comes out clean. 6. While the cupcakes are baking, make the glaze by combining the lemon juice and powdered sugar in a small bowl. Stir until smooth, then set aside. 7. Set the cupcakes aside to cool in the pans for about 5 minutes, then remove the cupcakes from the pans and transfer to a wire rack to cool completely. 8. Drizzle the glaze over the cooled cupcakes. Store in the refrigerator for up to 4 days.

Per Serving
Calories 227 | Total fat 13g | Saturated fat 2g | Carbohydrate 25g | Protein 3g

Dark Chocolate Bark with Fruit and Nuts

Prep timePrep Time: 15 minutes | Cook Time: 0 minutes | Serves 2

2 tablespoons chopped nuts (almonds, pecans, walnuts, hazelnuts, pistachios, or any combination of those)
3 ounces (85 g) good-quality dark chocolate chips (about ⅔ cup)
¼ cup chopped dried fruit (apricots, blueberries, figs, prunes, or any combination of those)

1. Line a sheet pan with parchment paper. 2. Place the nuts in a skillet over medium-high heat and toast them for 60 seconds, or just until they're fragrant. 3. Place the chocolate in a microwave-safe glass bowl or measuring cup and microwave on high for 1 minute. Stir the chocolate and allow any unmelted chips to warm and melt. If necessary, heat for another 20 to 30 seconds, but keep a close eye on it to make sure it doesn't burn. 4. Pour the chocolate onto the sheet pan. Sprinkle the dried fruit and nuts over the chocolate evenly and gently pat in so they stick. 5. Transfer the sheet pan to the refrigerator for at least 1 hour to let the chocolate harden. 6. When solid, break into pieces. Store any leftover chocolate in the refrigerator or freezer.

Per Serving
Calories: 284 | Total fat: 16g | Total carbs: 39g | Fiber: 2g | Sugar: 31g | Protein: 4g | Sodium: 2mg | Cholesterol: 0mg

Greek Yogurt with Honey and Pomegranates

Prep time: 5 minutes | Cook time: 0 minutes | Serves 4

4 cups plain full-fat Greek yogurt
¼ cup honey
½ cup pomegranate seeds
Sugar, for topping (optional)

1. Evenly divide the yogurt among four bowls. Evenly divide the pomegranate seeds among the bowls and drizzle each with the honey. 2. Sprinkle each bowl with a pinch of sugar, if desired, and serve.

Per Serving
Calories: 232 | Total fat: 8g | Total carbs: 33g | Sugar: 32g | Protein: 9g | Fiber: 1g | Sodium: 114mg

Individual Meringues with Strawberries, Mint, and Toasted Coconut

Prep time: 25 minutes | Cook time: 1 hour 30 minutes | Serves 6

4 large egg whites
½ teaspoon cream of tartar
8 ounces (227 g) strawberries, diced
¼ cup unsweetened shredded coconut, toasted

1 teaspoon vanilla extract
¾ cup sugar
¼ cup fresh mint, chopped

1. Preheat the oven to 225°F (107°C). Line 2 baking sheets with parchment paper. 2. Place the egg whites, vanilla, and cream of tartar in the bowl of a stand mixer (or use a large bowl with an electric hand mixer); beat at medium speed until soft peaks form, about 2 to 3 minutes. Increase to high speed and gradually add the sugar, beating until stiff peaks form and the mixture looks shiny and smooth, about 2 to 3 minutes. 3. Using a spatula or spoon, drop ⅓ cup of meringue onto a prepared baking sheet; smooth out and make shapelier as desired. In total, make 12 dollops, 6 per sheet, leaving at least 1 inch between dollops. 4. Bake for 1½ hours, rotating baking sheets between top and bottom, front and back, halfway through. After 1½ hours, turn off the oven, but keep the door closed. Leave the meringues in the oven for an additional 30 minutes. You can leave the meringues in the oven even longer (or overnight), or you may let them finish cooling to room temperature. 5. Combine the strawberries, mint, and coconut in a medium bowl. Serve 2 meringues per person topped with the fruit mixture.

Per Serving
Calories: 150 | Fat: 2g | Protein: 3g | Carbs: 29g | Sugars: 27g | Fiber: 1g | Sodium: 40mg | Cholesterol: 0mg

Crispy Apple Phyllo Tart

Prep time: 15 minutes | Cook time: 30 minutes | Serves 4

5 teaspoons extra virgin olive oil
¼ teaspoons ground cinnamon
1 large apple (any variety), peeled and cut into ⅛-inch (3mm) thick slices
1½ teaspoons apricot jam

2 teaspoons fresh lemon juice
1½ teaspoons granulated sugar, divided
5 (14 x 18-in/35.5 x 46cm) phyllo sheets, defrosted
1 teaspoon all-purpose flour

1. Preheat the oven to 350°F (177°C). Line a baking sheet with parchment paper, and pour the olive oil into a small dish. Set aside. 2. In a separate small bowl, combine the lemon juice, cinnamon, 1 teaspoon of the sugar, and the apple slices. Mix well to ensure the apple slices are coated in the seasonings. Set aside. 3. On a clean working surface, stack the phyllo sheets one on top of the other. Place a large bowl with an approximate diameter of 15 inches (38cm) on top of the sheets, then draw a sharp knife around the edge of the bowl to cut out a circle through all 5 sheets. Discard the remaining phyllo. 4. Working quickly, place the first sheet on the lined baking sheet and then brush with the olive oil. Repeat the process by placing a second sheet on top of the first sheet, then brushing the second sheet with olive oil. Repeat until all the phyllo sheets are in a single stack. 5. Sprinkle the flour and remaining sugar over the top of the sheets. Arrange the apples in overlapping circles 4 inches (10cm) from the edge of the phyllo. 6. Fold the edges of the phyllo in and then twist them all around the apple filling to form a crust edge. Brush the edge with the remaining olive oil. Bake for 30 minutes or until the crust is golden and the apples are browned on the edges. 7. While the tart is baking, heat the apricot jam in a small sauce pan over low heat until it's melted. 8. When the tart is done baking, brush the apples with the jam sauce. Slice the tart into 4 equal servings and serve warm. Store at room temperature, covered in plastic wrap, for up to 2 days.

Per Serving
Calories: 259 | Total fat: 18g | Saturated fat: 3g | Carbohydrate: 23g | Protein: 2g

Red Wine–Poached Figs with Ricotta and Almond

Prep time: 5 minutes | Cook time: 1 minute | Serves 4

2 cups water
¼ cup honey
1 star anise
12 dried mission figs
1 tablespoon confectioners' sugar
1 cup toasted sliced almonds

2 cups red wine
1 cinnamon stick
1 teaspoon vanilla bean paste
1 cup ricotta cheese
¼ teaspoon almond extract

1. Add water, wine, honey, cinnamon, star anise, and vanilla to the Instant Pot® and whisk well. Add figs, close lid, set steam release to Sealing, press the Manual button, and set time to 1 minute. 2. When the timer beeps, quick-release the pressure until the float valve drops. Press the Cancel button and open lid. With a slotted spoon, transfer figs to a plate and set aside to cool for 5 minutes. 3. In a small bowl, mix together ricotta, sugar, and almond extract. Serve figs with a dollop of sweetened ricotta and a sprinkling of almonds.

Per Serving
Calories: 597 | Fat: 21g | Protein: 13g | Sodium: 255mg | Fiber: 9 | Carbohydrates: 56g | Sugar: 37g

Ricotta-Lemon Cheesecake

Prep time: 5 minutes | Cook time: 1 hour | Serves 8 to 10

2 (8 ounces / 227 g)) packages full-fat cream cheese
1½ cups granulated sugar
5 large eggs

1 (16 ounces / 454 g) container full-fat ricotta cheese
1 tablespoon lemon zest
Nonstick cooking spray

1. Preheat the oven to 350ºF (177ºC). 2. Using a mixer, blend together the cream cheese and ricotta cheese. 3. Blend in the sugar and lemon zest. 4. Blend in the eggs; drop in 1 egg at a time, blend for 10 seconds, and repeat. 5. Line a 9-inch springform pan with parchment paper and nonstick spray. Wrap the bottom of the pan with foil. Pour the cheesecake batter into the pan. 6. To make a water bath, get a baking or roasting pan larger than the cheesecake pan. Fill the roasting pan about ⅓ of the way up with warm water. Put the cheesecake pan into the water bath. Put the whole thing in the oven and let the cheesecake bake for 1 hour. 7. After baking is complete, remove the cheesecake pan from the water bath and remove the foil. Let the cheesecake cool for 1 hour on the countertop. Then put it in the fridge to cool for at least 3 hours before serving.

Per Serving
Calories: 489 | Protein: 15g | Total Carbohydrates: 42g | Sugars: 40g | Fiber: 0g | Total Fat: 31g | Saturated Fat: 17g | Cholesterol: 210mg | Sodium: 264mg

Creamy Rice Pudding

Prep time: 5 minutes | Cook time: 45 minutes | Serves 6

1¼ cups long-grain rice
1 cup sugar
1 teaspoon cinnamon

5 cups whole milk
1 tablespoon rose water or orange blossom water

1. Rinse the rice under cold water for 30 seconds. 2. Put the rice, milk, and sugar in a large pot. Bring to a gentle boil while continually stirring. 3. Turn the heat down to low and let simmer for 40 to 45 minutes, stirring every 3 to 4 minutes so that the rice does not stick to the bottom of the pot. 4. Add the rose water at the end and simmer for 5 minutes. 5. Divide the pudding into 6 bowls. Sprinkle the top with cinnamon. Cool for at least 1 hour before serving. Store in the fridge.

Per Serving
Calories: 394 | Protein: 9g | Total Carbohydrates: 75g | Sugars: 43g | Fiber: 1g | Total Fat: 7g | Saturated Fat: 4g | Cholesterol: 29mg | Sodium: 102mg

Fruit Compote

Prep time: 15 minutes | Cook time: 11 minutes | Serves 6

- 1 cup apple juice
- 2 tablespoons honey
- ¼ teaspoon ground nutmeg
- 1½ tablespoons grated orange zest
- 3 large pears, peeled, cored, and chopped
- 1 cup dry white wine
- 1 cinnamon stick
- 1 tablespoon grated lemon zest
- 3 large apples, peeled, cored, and chopped
- ½ cup dried cherries

1. Place all ingredients in the Instant Pot® and stir well. Close lid, set steam release to Sealing, press the Manual button, and set time to 1 minute. When the timer beeps, quick-release the pressure until the float valve drops. Press the Cancel button and open lid. 2. Use a slotted spoon to transfer fruit to a serving bowl. Remove and discard cinnamon stick. Press the Sauté button and bring juice in the pot to a boil. Cook, stirring constantly, until reduced to a syrup that will coat the back of a spoon, about 10 minutes. 3. Stir syrup into fruit mixture. Allow to cool slightly, then cover with plastic wrap and refrigerate overnight.

Per Serving
Calories: 211 | Fat: 1g | Protein: 2g | Sodium: 7mg | Fiber: 5 | Carbohydrates: 44g | Sugar: 36g

Lightened-Up Baklava Rolls

Prep time: 2 minutes | Cook time: 1 hour 15 minutes | Serves 12

- 4 ounces (115g) shelled walnuts
- 1½ teaspoons granulated sugar
- 1 teaspoon extra virgin olive oil plus 2 tablespoons for brushing

For the syrup:
- ¼ cup water
- 1½ tablespoons fresh lemon juice
- 1¼ teaspoons ground cinnamon
- 5 teaspoons unseasoned breadcrumbs
- 6 (14 x 18-in/35.5 x 46cm) phyllo sheets, defrosted

- ½ cup granulated sugar

1. Preheat the oven to 350°F (177°C). 2. Make the syrup by combining the water and sugar in a small pan placed over medium heat. Bring to a boil, cook for 2 minutes, then remove the pan from the heat. Add the lemon juice, and stir. Set aside to cool. 3. In a food processor, combine the walnuts, cinnamon, sugar, breadcrumbs, and 1 teaspoon of the olive oil. Pulse until combined and grainy, but not chunky. 4. Place 1 phyllo sheet on a clean working surface and brush with the olive oil. Place a second sheet on top of the first sheet, brush with olive oil, and repeat the process with a third sheet. Cut the sheets in half crosswise, and then cut each half into 3 pieces crosswise. 5. Scatter 1 tablespoon of the walnut mixture over the phyllo sheet. Start rolling the phyllo and filling into a log shape while simultaneously folding the sides in (like a burrito) until the filling is encased in each piece of dough. The rolls should be about 3½ inches long. Place the rolls one next to the other in a large baking pan, then repeat the process with the remaining 3 phyllo sheets. You should have a total of 12 rolls. 6. Lightly brush the rolls with the remaining olive oil. Place in the oven to bake for 30 minutes or until the rolls turn golden brown, then remove from the oven and promptly drizzle the cold syrup over the top. 7. Let the rolls sit for 20 minutes, then flip them over and let them sit for an additional 20 minutes. Turn them over once more and sprinkle any remining walnut mixture over the rolls before serving. Store uncovered at room temperature for 2 days (to retain crispiness) and then cover with plastic wrap and store at room temperature for up to 10 days.

Per Serving
Calories: 133 | Total fat: 9g | Saturated fat: 1g | Carbohydrate: 12g | Protein: 8g

Cinnamon-Stewed Dried Plums with Greek Yogurt

Prep time: 5 minutes | Cook time: 3 minutes | Serves 6

3 cups dried plums
2 tablespoons sugar
3 cups low-fat plain Greek yogurt
2 cups water
2 cinnamon sticks

1. Add dried plums, water, sugar, and cinnamon to the Instant Pot®. Close lid, set steam release to Sealing, press the Manual button, and set time to 3 minutes. 2. When the timer beeps, quick-release the pressure until the float valve drops. Press the Cancel button and open lid. Remove and discard cinnamon sticks. Serve warm over Greek yogurt.

Per Serving
Calories: 301 | Fat: 2g | Protein: 14g | Sodium: 50mg | Fiber: 4 | Carbohydrates: 61g | Sugar: 33g

Chocolate Hazelnut "Powerhouse" Truffles

Prep time: 5 minutes | Cook time: 50 minutes | Makes 12 truffles

Filling
1¾ cups (236 g/8.3 ounces) blanched hazelnuts, divided
virgin coconut oil
¼ cup (22 g/0.8 ounces) raw cacao powder
Optional: low-carb sweetener, to taste
2.5 ounces (75 g) 100% dark chocolate
Pinch of salt
½ cup (125 g/4.4 ounces) coconut butter
4 tablespoons (57 g/2 ounces) butter or ¼ cup (60 ml)
¼ cup (25 g/0.9 ounces) collagen powder
1 teaspoon vanilla powder or cinnamon
Chocolate coating
1 ounce (28 g) cacao butter

1. Preheat the oven to 285°F (140°C) fan assisted or 320°F (160°C) conventional. 2. To make the filling: Spread the hazelnuts on a baking tray and roast for 40 to 50 minutes, until lightly golden. Remove from the oven and let cool for a few minutes. 3. Place 1 cup (136 g/4.8 ounces) of the roasted hazelnuts in a food processor. Process for 1 to 2 minutes, until chunky. Add the coconut butter, butter, collagen powder, cacao powder, vanilla, and sweetener, if using. Process again until well combined. Place the dough in the fridge to set for 1 hour. 4. Reserve 12 hazelnuts for filling and crumble the remaining hazelnuts unto small pieces. 5. To make the chocolate coating: Line a baking tray with parchment. Melt the dark chocolate and cacao butter in a double boiler, or use a heatproof bowl placed over a small saucepan filled with 1 cup (240 ml) of water, placed over medium heat. Remove from the heat and let cool to room temperature before using for coating. Alternatively, use a microwave and melt in short 10- to 15-second bursts until melted, stirring in between. 6. Remove the dough from the fridge and use a spoon to scoop about 1 ounce (28 g) of the dough. Press one whole hazelnut into the center and use your hands to wrap the dough around to create a truffle. Place in the freezer for about 15 minutes. 7. Gently pierce each very cold truffle with a toothpick or a fork. Working one at a time, hold the truffle over the melted chocolate and spoon the chocolate over it to coat completely. Turn the toothpick as you work until the coating is solidified. Place the coated truffles on the lined tray and drizzle any remaining coating over them. Before they become completely solid, roll them in the chopped nuts. Refrigerate the coated truffles for at least 15 minutes to harden. 8. Keep refrigerated for up to 1 week or freeze for up to 3 months.

Per Serving
Total carbs: 7.4 g | Fiber: 4.5 g | Net Carbs: 2.9 g | Protein: 6.6 g | Fat: 27.9 g (of which saturated: 13.1 g) | Calories: 283 kcal

Strawberry-Pomegranate Molasses Sauce

Prep time: 10 minutes | Cook time: 5 minutes | Serves 6

3 tablespoons olive oil
2 pints strawberries, hulled and halved
2 tablespoons chopped fresh mint
¼ cup honey
1 to 2 tablespoons pomegranate molasses
Greek yogurt, for serving

1. In a medium saucepan, heat the olive oil over medium heat. Add the strawberries; cook until their juices are released. Stir in the honey and cook for 1 to 2 minutes. Stir in the molasses and mint. Serve warm over Greek yogurt.

Per Serving
Calories: 189 | Fat: 7g | Protein: 4g | Carbs: 24g | Sugars: 20g | Fiber: 3g | Sodium: 12mg | Cholesterol: 10mg

Greek Yogurt Ricotta Mousse

Prep time: 1 hour 5 minutes | Cook time: 0 minutes | Serves 4

9 ounces (250g) full-fat ricotta cheese
3 teaspoons fresh lemon juice
2 tablespoons granulated sugar
4.5 ounces (125g) 2% Greek yogurt
½ teaspoons pure vanilla extract

1. Combine all of the ingredients in a food processor. Blend until smooth, about 1 minute. 2. Divide the mousse between 4 serving glasses. Cover and transfer to the refrigerator to chill for 1 hour before serving. Store covered in the refrigerator for up to 4 days.

Per Serving
Calories: 159 | Total fat: 9g | Saturated fat: 6g | Carbohydrate: 10g | Protein: 10g

Blueberry Compote

Prep time: 10 minutes | Cook time: 5 minutes | Serves 8

1 (16 ounces / 454 g) bag frozen blueberries, thawed
1 tablespoon lemon juice
2 tablespoons water
¼ teaspoon grated lemon zest
¼ cup sugar
2 tablespoons cornstarch
¼ teaspoon vanilla extract

1. Add blueberries, sugar, and lemon juice to the Instant Pot®. Close lid, set steam release to Sealing, press the Manual button, and set time to 1 minute. 2. When the timer beeps, quick-release the pressure until the float valve drops. Press the Cancel button and open lid. 3. Press the Sauté button. In a small bowl, combine cornstarch and water. Stir into blueberry mixture and cook until mixture comes to a boil and thickens, about 3–4 minutes. Press the Cancel button and stir in vanilla and lemon zest. Serve immediately or refrigerate until ready to serve.

Per Serving
Calories: 57 | Fat: 0g | Protein: 0g | Sodium: 0mg | Fiber: 2g | Carbohydrates: 14g | Sugar: 7g

Figs with Mascarpone and Honey

Prep time: 5 minutes | Cook time: 5 minutes | Serves 4

- ⅓ cup walnuts, chopped
- ¼ cup mascarpone cheese
- ¼ teaspoon flaked sea salt
- 8 fresh figs, halved
- 1 tablespoon honey

1. In a skillet over medium heat, toast the walnuts, stirring often, 3 to 5 minutes. 2. Arrange the figs cut-side up on a plate or platter. Using your finger, make a small depression in the cut side of each fig and fill with mascarpone cheese. Sprinkle with a bit of the walnuts, drizzle with the honey, and add a tiny pinch of sea salt.

Per Serving
Calories: 200 | Fat: 13g | Protein: 3g | Carbs: 24g | Sugars: 18g | Fiber: 3g | Sodium: 105mg | Cholesterol: 18mg

Spiced Baked Pears with Mascarpone

Prep timePrep Time: 10 minutes | Cook Time: 20 minutes | Serves 2

- 2 ripe pears, peeled
- 1 teaspoon vanilla, divided
- ¼ teaspoon ground coriander
- ¼ cup mascarpone cheese
- 1 tablespoon plus 2 teaspoons honey, divided
- ¼ teaspoon ginger
- ¼ cup minced walnuts
- Pinch salt

1. Preheat the oven to 350°F (177°C) and set the rack to the middle position. Grease a small baking dish. 2. Cut the pears in half lengthwise. Using a spoon, scoop out the core from each piece. Place the pears with the cut side up in the baking dish. 3. Combine 1 tablespoon of honey, ½ teaspoon of vanilla, ginger, and coriander in a small bowl. Pour this mixture evenly over the pear halves. 4. Sprinkle walnuts over the pear halves. 5. Bake for 20 minutes, or until the pears are golden and you're able to pierce them easily with a knife. 6. While the pears are baking, mix the mascarpone cheese with the remaining 2 teaspoons honey, ½ teaspoon of vanilla, and a pinch of salt. Stir well to combine. 7. Divide the mascarpone among the warm pear halves and serve.

Per Serving
Calories: 307 | Total fat: 16g | Total carbs: 43g | Fiber: 6g | Sugar: 31g | Protein: 4g | Sodium: 89mg | Cholesterol: 18mg

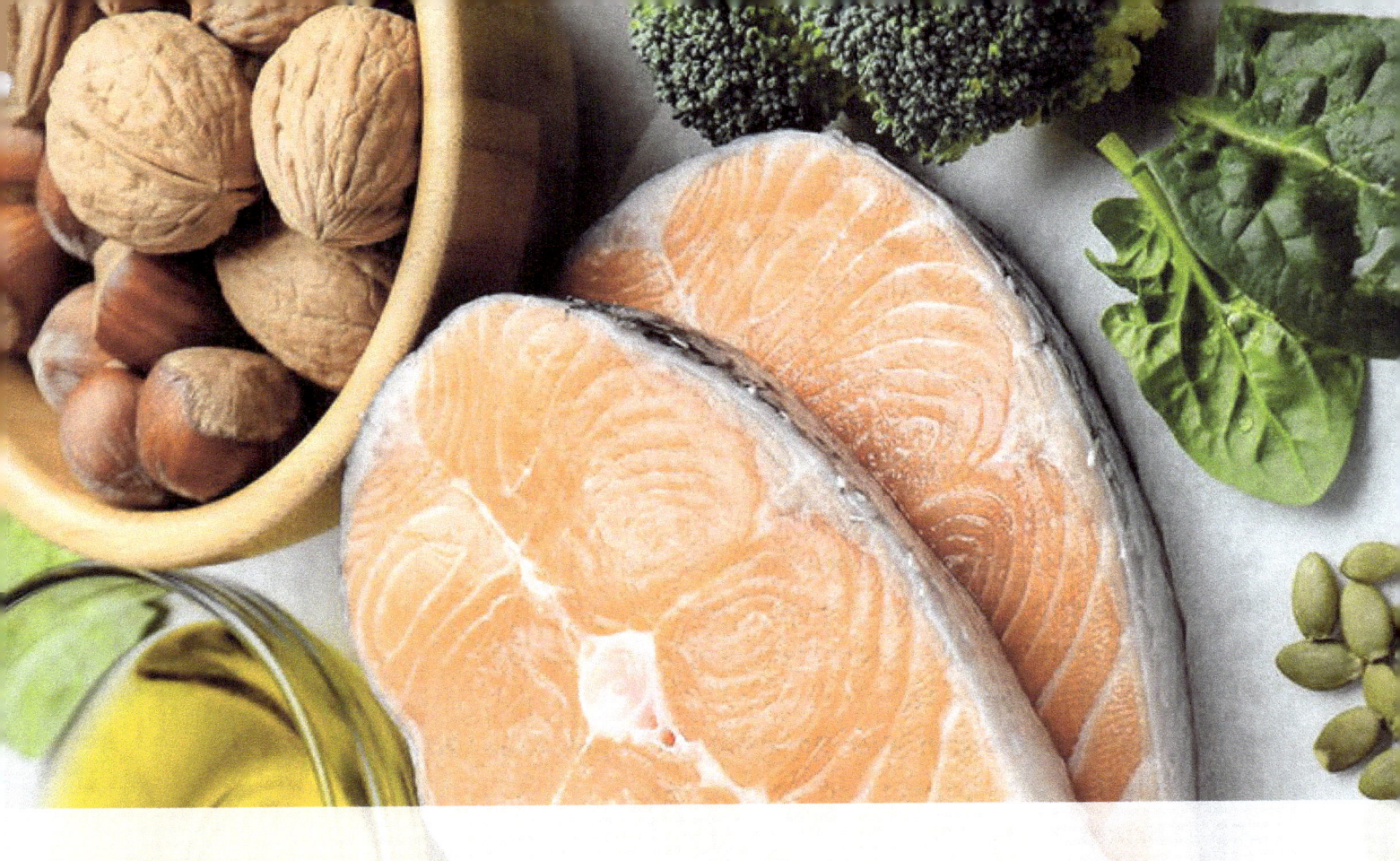

Chapter 6   Fish and Seafood

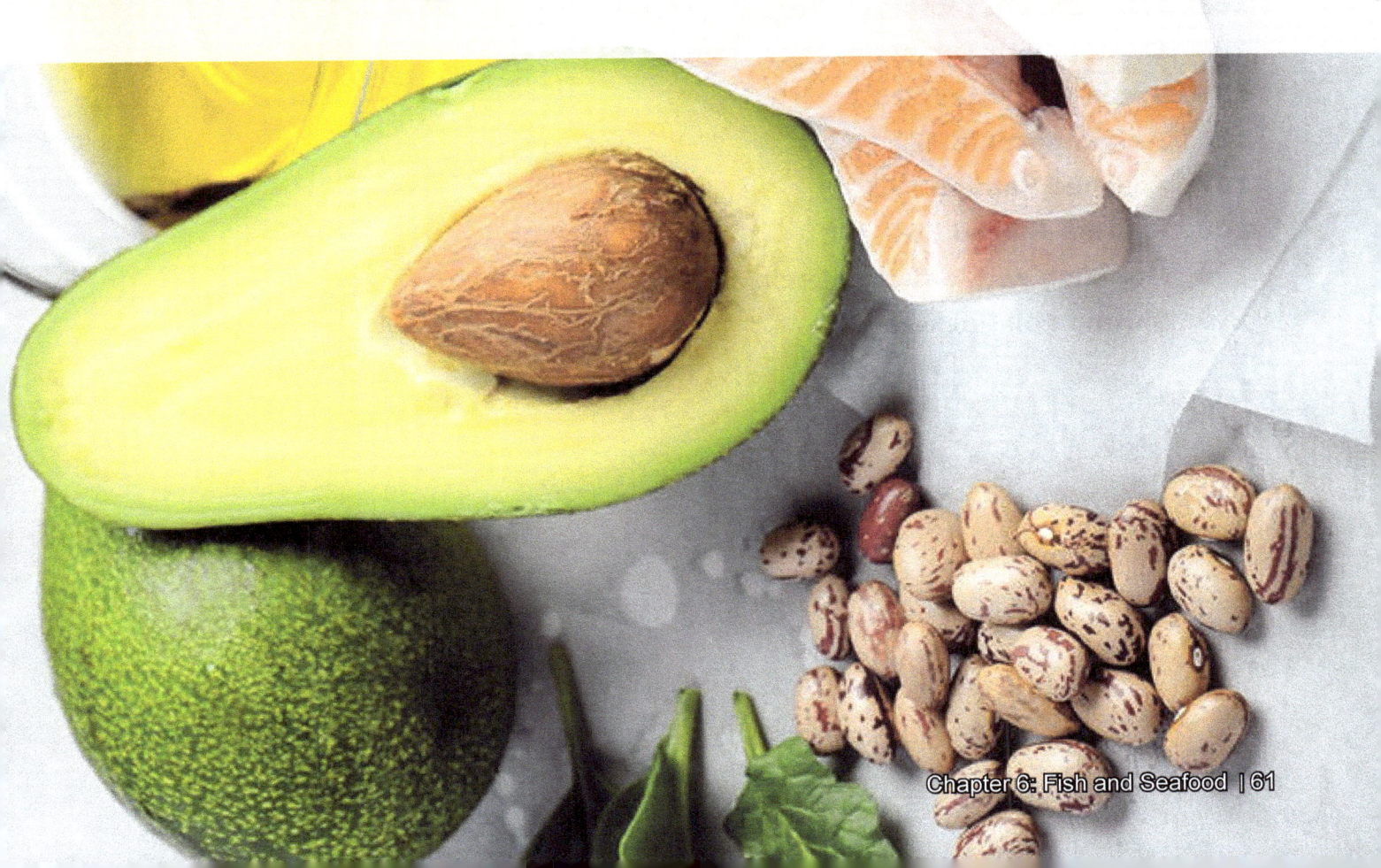

87	Shrimp Pasta with Basil and Mushrooms	63
88	Hake in Saffron Broth	63
89	Easy Shrimp Paella	64
90	Pesto Shrimp with Wild Rice Pilaf	64
91	Italian Breaded Shrimp	64
92	Herbed Tuna Steaks	65
93	Seasoned Tuna Steaks	65
94	Baked Salmon and Tomato Pockets	65
95	Shrimp and Asparagus Risotto	66
96	Mediterranean Garlic and Herb-Roasted Cod	66
97	Poached Octopus	67
98	Baked Red Snapper with Potatoes and Tomatoes	67
99	Whitefish with Lemon and Capers	68
100	Shrimp Paella	68
101	Lemon Salmon with Dill	68
102	Flounder with Tomatoes and Basil	69
103	Sea Bass with Roasted Root Vegetables	69
104	Salmon with Tarragon-Dijon Sauce	69
105	Greek Fish Pitas	70
106	Italian Baccalà	70
107	Poached Salmon	70
108	Paprika-Spiced Fish	71
109	Monkfish with Sautéed Leeks, Fennel, and Tomatoes	71
110	Shrimp Foil Packets	71

Shrimp Pasta with Basil and Mushrooms

Prep time: 10 minutes | Cook time: 10 minutes | Serves 6

1 pound (454 g) small shrimp, peeled and deveined
¼ teaspoon garlic powder
1 pound (454 g) whole grain pasta
8 ounces (227 g) baby bella mushrooms, sliced
1 teaspoon salt
½ cup fresh basil
¼ cup plus 1 tablespoon olive oil, divided
¼ teaspoon cayenne
5 garlic cloves, minced
½ cup Parmesan, plus more for serving (optional)
½ teaspoon black pepper

1. Preheat the air fryer to 380°F (193°C). 2. In a small bowl, combine the shrimp, 1 tablespoon olive oil, garlic powder, and cayenne. Toss to coat the shrimp. 3. Place the shrimp into the air fryer basket and roast for 5 minutes. Remove the shrimp and set aside. 4. Cook the pasta according to package directions. Once done cooking, reserve ½ cup pasta water, then drain. 5. Meanwhile, in a large skillet, heat ¼ cup of olive oil over medium heat. Add the garlic and mushrooms and cook down for 5 minutes. 6. Pour the pasta, reserved pasta water, Parmesan, salt, pepper, and basil into the skillet with the vegetable-and-oil mixture, and stir to coat the pasta. 7. Toss in the shrimp and remove from heat, then let the mixture sit for 5 minutes before serving with additional Parmesan, if desired.

Per Serving
Calories: 457 | Total Fat: 15g | Saturated Fat: 3g | Protein: 25g | Total Carbohydrates: 60g | Fiber: 7g | Sugar: 1g | Cholesterol: 100mg

Hake in Saffron Broth

Prep time: 15 minutes | Cook time: 10 minutes | Serves 4

2 tablespoons extra-virgin olive oil, divided, plus extra for drizzling
4 garlic cloves, minced
1 (8 ounces / 227 g)) bottle clam juice
½ cup dry white wine
¼ teaspoon saffron threads, crumbled
4 (6 ounces / 170 g) skinless hake fillets, 1½ inches thick
2 tablespoons minced fresh parsley
1 onion, chopped
4 ounces (113 g) Spanish-style chorizo sausage, sliced ¼ inch thick
¾ cup water
8 ounces (227 g) small red potatoes, unpeeled, quartered
1 bay leaf
½ teaspoon table salt
¼ teaspoon pepper

1. Using highest sauté function, heat 1 tablespoon oil in Instant Pot until shimmering. Add onion and chorizo and cook until onion is softened and lightly browned, 5 to 7 minutes. Stir in garlic and cook until fragrant, about 30 seconds. Stir in clam juice, water, and wine, scraping up any browned bits. Turn off Instant Pot, then stir in potatoes, saffron, and bay leaf. 2. Fold sheet of aluminum foil into 16 by 6-inch sling. Brush hake with remaining 1 tablespoon oil and sprinkle with salt and pepper. Arrange hake skinned side down in center of sling. Using sling, lower hake into Instant Pot on top of potato mixture;
allow narrow edges of sling to rest along sides of insert. Lock lid in place and close pressure release valve. Select high pressure cook function and cook for 3 minutes. 3. Turn off Instant Pot and quick-release pressure. Carefully remove lid, allowing steam to escape away from you. Using sling, transfer hake to large plate. Tent with aluminum foil and let rest while finishing potato mixture. 4. Discard bay leaf. Stir parsley into potato mixture and season with salt to taste. Serve cod with potato mixture and broth, drizzling individual portions with extra oil.

Per Serving
Cal: 410 | Total Fat: 19g | Sat Fat: 5g | Chol: 100mg | Sodium: 880mg | Total Carbs: 14g, Fiber: 2g, Total Sugar: 2g | Added Sugar: 0g | Protein: 39g

Easy Shrimp Paella

Prep timePrep Time: 20 minutes | Cook Time: 1 hour 5 minutes | Serves 2

2 tablespoons olive oil
1 garlic clove, minced
1 cup diced tomato (about 1 medium tomato)
Generous pinch saffron
½ cup dry white wine
8 ounces (227 g) large raw shrimp
¼ cup jarred roasted red peppers, cut into strips (about 1 whole pepper)
½ large onion, minced
4 ounces (113 g) chorizo sausage, removed from casing
½ teaspoon sweet paprika
½ cup medium- or short-grain rice
1¼ cups low-sodium chicken stock
1 cup frozen peas
Salt

1. Heat the olive oil in a large sauté pan over medium-high heat. Add the onion, garlic, and chorizo, and sauté for 10 minutes, or until the onion is wilted and the chorizo is cooked. 2. Add the tomato, paprika, saffron, and rice, and stir for 3 minutes to toast the rice and spices. 3. Add the wine and chicken stock and stir. Bring the mixture to a boil. Cover and reduce the heat to medium-low, and let the paella cook for 45 minutes, or until the rice is just about tender and most, but not all, of the liquid has been absorbed. 4. Add the shrimp, peas, and roasted red peppers. Cover and cook for another 5 minutes. Season with salt.

Per Serving
Calories: 645 | Total fat: 27g | Total carbs: 60g | Fiber: 7g | Sugar: 9g | Protein: 42g | Sodium: 686mg | Cholesterol: 262mg

Pesto Shrimp with Wild Rice Pilaf

Prep time: 5 minutes | Cook time: 5 minutes | Serves 4

1 pound (454 g) medium shrimp, peeled and deveined
1 lemon, sliced
¼ cup pesto sauce
2 cups cooked wild rice pilaf

1. Preheat the air fryer to 360ºF (182°C). 2. In a medium bowl, toss the shrimp with the pesto sauce until well coated. 3. Place the shrimp in a single layer in the air fryer basket. Put the lemon slices over the shrimp and roast for 5 minutes. 4. Remove the lemons and discard. Serve a quarter of the shrimp over ½ cup wild rice with some favorite steamed vegetables.

Per Serving
Calories: 249 | Total Fat: 10g | Saturated Fat: 2g | Protein: 20g | Total Carbohydrates: 20g | Fiber: 2g | Sugar: 1g | Cholesterol: 145mg

Italian Breaded Shrimp

Prep time: 10 minutes | Cook time: 5 minutes | Serves 4

2 large eggs
1 teaspoon salt
1 pound (454 g) large shrimp (21-25), peeled and deveined
2 cups seasoned Italian breadcrumbs
1 cup flour
Extra-virgin olive oil

1. In a small bowl, beat the eggs with 1 tablespoon water, then transfer to a shallow dish. 2. Add the breadcrumbs and salt to a separate shallow dish; mix well. 3. Place the flour into a third shallow dish. 4. Coat the shrimp in the flour, then egg, and finally the breadcrumbs. Place on a plate and repeat with all of the shrimp. 5. Preheat a skillet over high heat. Pour in enough olive oil to coat the bottom of the skillet. Cook the shrimp in the hot skillet for 2 to 3 minutes on each side. Take the shrimp out and drain on a paper towel. Serve warm.

Per Serving
Calories: 714 | Protein: 37g | Total Carbohydrates: 63g | Sugars: 4g | Fiber: 3g | Total Fat: 34g | Saturated Fat: 4g | Cholesterol: 243mg | Sodium: 1,727mg

Herbed Tuna Steaks

Prep time: 10 minutes | Cook time: 4 to 6 hours | Serves 4

Nonstick cooking spray
1 teaspoon sea salt
¼ teaspoon freshly ground black pepper
2 teaspoons dried thyme
4 (1-inch-thick) fresh tuna steaks (about 2 pounds (907g) total)
2 teaspoons extra-virgin olive oil
2 teaspoons dried rosemary

1. Coat a slow-cooker insert with cooking spray, or line the bottom and sides with parchment paper or aluminum foil. 2. Season the tuna steaks all over with salt and pepper and place them in the prepared slow cooker in a single layer. Drizzle with the olive oil and sprinkle with the thyme and rosemary. 3. Cover the cooker and cook for 4 to 6 hours on Low heat.

Per Serving
Calories: 339 | Total fat: 5g | Sodium: 689mg | Carbohydrates: 1g | Fiber: 1g | Sugar: 0g | Protein: 68g

Seasoned Tuna Steaks

Prep time: 5 minutes | Cook time: 9 minutes | Serves 4

1 teaspoon garlic powder
¼ teaspoon dried thyme
4 tuna steaks
1 lemon, quartered
½ teaspoon salt
¼ teaspoon dried oregano
2 tablespoons olive oil

1. Preheat the air fryer to 380°F (193°C). 2. In a small bowl, whisk together the garlic powder, salt, thyme, and oregano. 3. Coat the tuna steaks with olive oil. Season both sides of each steak with the seasoning blend. Place the steaks in a single layer in the air fryer basket. 4. Roast for 5 minutes, then flip and roast for an additional 3 to 4 minutes.

Per Serving
Calories: 269 | Total Fat: 14g | Saturated Fat: 3g | Protein: 33g | Total Carbohydrates: 1g | Fiber: 0g | Sugar: 0g | Cholesterol: 54mg

Baked Salmon and Tomato Pockets

Prep time: 5 minutes | Cook time: 25 minutes | Serves 4

1 pint (2 cups) cherry tomatoes
3 tablespoons lemon juice
3 tablespoons unsalted butter, melted
4 (5 ounces / 142 g) salmon fillets
3 tablespoons extra-virgin olive oil
1 teaspoon oregano
½ teaspoon salt

1. Preheat the oven to 400°F (204°C). 2. Cut the tomatoes in half and put them in a bowl. 3. Add the olive oil, lemon juice, oregano, melted butter, and salt to the tomatoes and toss to combine. 4. Cut 4 pieces of foil, about 12-by-12 inches each. 5. Place the salmon in the middle of each piece of foil. 6. Divide the tomato mixture evenly over the 4 pieces of salmon. Bring the ends of the foil together and seal to form a closed pocket. 7. Place the 4 pockets on a baking sheet. Cook for 25 minutes. 8. To serve, place each pocket on a plate and let your guests open to reveal the baked salmon and tomatoes.

Per Serving
Calories: 410 | Protein: 30g | Total Carbohydrates: 4g | Sugars: 2g | Fiber: 1g | Total Fat: 32g | Saturated Fat: 9g | Cholesterol: 80mg | Sodium: 370mg

Shrimp and Asparagus Risotto

Prep time: 15 minutes | Cook time: 20 minutes | Serves 4

¼ cup extra-virgin olive oil, divided
½ onion, chopped fine
¼ teaspoon table salt
3 garlic cloves, minced
3 cups chicken or vegetable broth, plus extra as needed
2 ounces Parmesan cheese, grated (1 cup)
1 tablespoon minced fresh chives
8 ounces (227 g) asparagus, trimmed and cut on bias into 1-inch lengths
1½ cups Arborio rice
½ cup dry white wine
1 pound (454 g) large shrimp (26 to 30 per pound), peeled and deveined
1 tablespoon lemon juice

1. Using highest sauté function, heat 1 tablespoon oil in Instant Pot until shimmering. Add asparagus, partially cover, and cook until just crisp-tender, about 4 minutes. Using slotted spoon, transfer asparagus to bowl; set aside. 2. Add onion, 2 tablespoons oil, and salt to now-empty pot and cook, using highest sauté function, until onion is softened, about 5 minutes. Stir in rice and garlic and cook until grains are translucent around edges, about 3 minutes. Stir in wine and cook until nearly evaporated, about 1 minute. 3. Stir in broth, scraping up any rice that sticks to bottom of pot. Lock lid in place and close pressure release valve. Select high pressure cook function and cook for 7 minutes. 4. Turn off Instant Pot and quick-release pressure. Carefully remove lid, allowing steam to escape away from you. Stir shrimp and asparagus into risotto, cover, and let sit until shrimp are opaque throughout, 5 to 7 minutes. Add Parmesan and remaining 1 tablespoon oil, and stir vigorously until risotto becomes creamy. Adjust consistency with extra hot broth as needed. Stir in lemon juice and season with salt and pepper to taste. 5. Sprinkle individual portions with chives before serving.

Per Serving
Cal: 540 | Total Fat: 21g | Sat Fat: 4g | Chol: 115mg | Sodium: 1310mg | Total Carbs: 58g, Fiber: 2g, Total Sugar: 2g | Added Sugar: 0g | Protein: 27g

Mediterranean Garlic and Herb-Roasted Cod

Prep time: 10 minutes | Cook time: 15 minutes | Serves 3

4½ tablespoons extra virgin olive oil plus 1 teaspoon for brushing
1½ teaspoons dried onion flakes
¼ teaspoons freshly ground black pepper
1 garlic clove, minced
1 pound (450g) cod fillets (about 3–4), patted dry
For the topping
4 tablespoons unseasoned breadcrumbs
1½ tablespoons dried oregano
1 teaspoon paprika
½ teaspoons salt
1½ tablespoons fresh lemon juice plus extra for serving
3 teaspoons Dijon mustard
2 tablespoons chopped fresh parsley
1½ tablespoons extra virgin olive oil

1. Preheat the oven to 430°F (220°C). Brush a baking dish large enough to hold the fish in a single layer with 1 teaspoon of the olive oil. 2. In a small bowl, combine the oregano, paprika, onion flakes, salt, and black pepper. Mix well and set aside. 3. In a medium bowl, combine 4½ tablespoons of the olive oil, lemon juice, garlic, and Dijon mustard. Add the dry ingredients to the wet ingredients and mix well. 4. Dip each fillet in the coating and toss to coat, then place the fillets in the dish and drizzle the leftover coating over the top of the fillets. 5. Make the breadcrumb topping by combining the breadcrumbs and olive oil in a small bowl and mixing with a fork. Sprinkle the breadcrumb mixture over the fillets. 6. Place in the oven and roast for 15 minutes or until the breadcrumb topping becomes golden brown. 7. Transfer to a plate and top with the chopped parsley and a squeeze of lemon. (This recipe is best eaten fresh.)

Per Serving
Calories: 403 | Total fat: 29g | Saturated fat: 4g | Carbohydrate: 11g | Protein: 24g

Poached Octopus

Prep time: 10 minutes | Cook time: 16 minutes | Serves 8

2 pounds (907g) potatoes (about 6 medium)
1 (2-pound) frozen octopus, thawed, cleaned, and rinsed
2 teaspoons whole peppercorns
¼ cup white wine vinegar
½ cup chopped fresh parsley
3 teaspoons salt, divided
3 cloves garlic, peeled, divided
1 bay leaf
½ cup olive oil
½ teaspoon ground black pepper

1. Place potatoes in the Instant Pot® with 2 teaspoons salt and enough water to just cover the potatoes halfway. Close lid, set steam release to Sealing, press the Manual button, and set time to 6 minutes. When the timer beeps, quick-release the pressure until the float valve drops and open lid. Press the Cancel button. 2. Remove potatoes with tongs (reserve the cooking water), and peel them as soon as you can handle them. Dice potatoes into bite-sized pieces. Set aside. 3. Add octopus to potato cooking water in the pot and add more water to cover if needed. Add 1 garlic clove, bay leaf, and peppercorns. Close lid, set steam release to Sealing, press the Manual button, and set time to 10 minutes. When the timer beeps, quick-release the pressure until the float valve drops and open lid. Remove and discard bay leaf. 4. Check octopus for tenderness by seeing if a fork will sink easily into the thickest part of the flesh. If not, close the top and bring it to pressure for another minute or two and check again. 5. Remove octopus and drain. Chop head and tentacles into small, bite-sized chunks. 6. Crush remaining 2 garlic cloves and place in a small jar or plastic container. Add olive oil, vinegar, remaining 1 teaspoon salt, and pepper. Close the lid and shake well. 7. In a large serving bowl, mix potatoes with octopus, cover with vinaigrette, and sprinkle with parsley.

Per Serving
Calories: 301 | Fat: 15g | Protein: 15g | Sodium: 883mg | Fiber: 2g | Carbohydrates: 30g | Sugar: 1g

Baked Red Snapper with Potatoes and Tomatoes

Prep time: 10 minutes | Cook time: 45 minutes | Serves 4

5 sprigs fresh thyme, divided
1½ pounds (680 g) new potatoes, halved (or quartered if large)
4 cloves garlic, halved, divided
¾ teaspoon ground black pepper, divided
½–1 lemon, sliced
4 cups (4 ounces / 113 g) baby spinach
2 sprigs fresh oregano, divided
4 Roma tomatoes, quartered lengthwise
1 tablespoon plus 1 teaspoon olive oil
1¼ teaspoons kosher salt, divided
1 cleaned whole red snapper (about 2 pounds (907g)), scaled and fins removed

1. Preheat the oven to 350°F (177°C). 2. Strip the leaves off 2 sprigs thyme and 1 sprig oregano and chop. In a 9' × 13' baking dish, toss the potatoes and tomatoes with 1 tablespoon of the oil, the chopped thyme and oregano leaves, 2 cloves of the garlic, 1 teaspoon of the salt, and ½ teaspoon of the pepper. 3. Cut 3 or 4 diagonal slashes in the skin on both sides of the snapper. Rub the skin with the remaining 1 teaspoon oil. Sprinkle the cavity of the snapper with the remaining ¼ teaspoon salt and pepper. Fill it with the lemon slices, the remaining thyme and oregano sprigs, and the remaining 2 cloves garlic. Sprinkle the outside of the snapper with a pinch of salt and pepper. Set the fish on the vegetables. 4. Cover the baking dish with foil and bake for 20 minutes. Remove the foil and continue baking until the potatoes are tender and the fish flakes easily with a fork, 20 to 25 minutes. 5. Transfer the fish to a serving platter. Toss the spinach with the tomatoes and potatoes in the baking dish, until wilted. 6. Using forks, peel the skin off the fish fillets. Scatter the vegetables around the fish and serve.

Per Serving
calories: 345 | protein: 39g | carbohydrates: 33g | sugars: 4g | total fat: 6g | saturated fat: 1g | fiber: 5g | sodium: 782mg

Whitefish with Lemon and Capers

Prep time: 5 minutes | Cook time: 20 minutes | Serves 4

- 4 (4- to 5 ounces / 113 g-142 g) cod fillets (or any whitefish)
- 4 tablespoons (½ stick) unsalted butter
- 3 tablespoons lemon juice
- 1 tablespoon extra-virgin olive oil
- 1 teaspoon salt, divided
- 2 tablespoons capers, drained
- ½ teaspoon freshly ground black pepper

1. Preheat the oven to 450°F (235°C). Put the cod in a large baking dish and drizzle with the olive oil and ½ teaspoon of salt. Bake for 15 minutes. 2. Right before the fish is done cooking, melt the butter in a small saucepan over medium heat. Add the capers, lemon juice, remaining ½ teaspoon of salt, and pepper; simmer for 30 seconds. 3. Place the fish in a serving dish once it is done baking; spoon the caper sauce over the fish and serve.

Per Serving

Calories: 255 | Protein: 26g | Total Carbohydrates: 1g | Sugars: 0g | Fiber: 0g | Total Fat: 16g | Saturated Fat: 8g | Cholesterol: 94mg | Sodium: 801mg

Shrimp Paella

Prep time: 10 minutes | Cook time: 25 minutes | Serves 4

- 2 tablespoons olive oil
- 1 red bell pepper, diced
- Pinch of saffron (about 8 threads)
- 1 teaspoon salt
- 3 cups chicken broth, divided
- 1 pound (454 g) peeled and deveined large shrimp
- 1 medium onion, diced
- 3 cloves garlic, minced
- ¼ teaspoon hot paprika
- ½ teaspoon freshly ground black pepper
- 1 cup short-grain white rice
- 1 cup frozen peas, thawed

1. Heat the oil in a wide, heavy skillet set over medium heat. Add the onion and bell pepper and cook, stirring frequently, until the vegetables are softened, about 6 minutes. Add the garlic, saffron, paprika, salt, and pepper and stir to mix. Stir in 2½ cups of broth, and the rice. 2. Bring the mixture to a boil, then lower the heat to low, cover, and simmer until the rice is nearly cooked through, about 12 minutes. Scatter the shrimp and peas over the rice and add the remaining ½ cup of broth. Place the lid back on the skillet and cook for about 5 minutes more, until the shrimp are just cooked through. Serve immediately.

Per Serving

Calories: 409 | Total Fat: 10g | Saturated Fat: 1g | Carbs: 51g | Protein: 25g | Sodium: 1,414mg | Fiber: 4g

Lemon Salmon with Dill

Prep time: 10 minutes | Cook time: 3 minutes | Serves 4

- 1 cup water
- ½ teaspoon salt
- ¼ cup chopped fresh dill
- 2 tablespoons extra-virgin olive oil
- 4 (4 ounces / 113 g) skin-on salmon fillets
- ½ teaspoon ground black pepper
- 1 small lemon, thinly sliced
- 1 tablespoon chopped fresh parsley

1. Add water to the Instant Pot® and place rack inside. 2. Season fish fillets with salt and pepper. Place fillets on rack. Top each fillet with dill and two or three lemon slices. Close lid, set steam release to Sealing, press the Steam button, and set time to 3 minutes. 3. When the timer beeps, quick-release the pressure until the float valve drops. Press the Cancel button and open lid. Place fillets on a serving platter, drizzle with olive oil, and garnish with parsley. Serve immediately.

Per Serving

Calories: 160 | Fat: 9g | Protein: 19g | Sodium: 545mg | Fiber: 0g | Carbohydrates: 0g | Sugar: 0g

Flounder with Tomatoes and Basil

Prep time: 10 minutes | Cook time: 20 minutes | Serves 4

1 pound (454 g) cherry tomatoes
2 tablespoons extra-virgin olive oil
2 tablespoons basil, cut into ribbons
¼ teaspoon freshly ground black pepper
4 garlic cloves, sliced
2 tablespoons lemon juice
½ teaspoon kosher salt
4 (5- to 6 ounces / 142- to 170-g) flounder fillets

1. Preheat the oven to 425°F (218°C). 2. In a baking dish, combine the tomatoes, garlic, olive oil, lemon juice, basil, salt, and black pepper; mix well. Bake for 5 minutes. 3. Remove the baking dish from the oven and arrange the flounder on top of the tomato mixture. Bake until the fish is opaque and begins to flake, about 10 to 15 minutes, depending on thickness.

Per Serving
Calories: 215 | Fat: 9g | Protein: 28g | Carbs: 6g | Sugars: 3g | Fiber: 2g | Sodium: 261mg | Cholesterol: 68mg

Sea Bass with Roasted Root Vegetables

Prep time: 10 minutes | Cook time: 15 minutes | Serves 4

1 carrot, diced small
1 rutabaga, diced small
2 teaspoons salt, divided
½ teaspoon onion powder
1 lemon, sliced, plus additional wedges for serving
1 parsnip, diced small
¼ cup olive oil
4 sea bass fillets
2 garlic cloves, minced

1. Preheat the air fryer to 380°F (193°C). 2. In a small bowl, toss the carrot, parsnip, and rutabaga with olive oil and 1 teaspoon salt. 3. Lightly season the sea bass with the remaining 1 teaspoon of salt and the onion powder, then place it into the air fryer basket in a single layer. 4. Spread the garlic over the top of each fillet, then cover with lemon slices. 5. Pour the prepared vegetables into the basket around and on top of the fish. Roast for 15 minutes. 6. Serve with additional lemon wedges if desired.

Per Serving
Calories: 299 | Total Fat: 16g | Saturated Fat: 3g | Protein: 25g | Total Carbohydrates: 13g | Fiber: 3g | Sugar: 5g | Cholesterol: 53mg

Salmon with Tarragon-Dijon Sauce

Prep time: 5 minutes | Cook time: 15 minutes | Serves 4

1¼ pounds (567 g) salmon fillet (skin on or removed), cut into 4 equal pieces
Zest and juice of ½ lemon
½ teaspoon salt
¼ teaspoon freshly ground black pepper
¼ cup avocado oil mayonnaise
¼ cup Dijon or stone-ground mustard
2 tablespoons chopped fresh tarragon or 1 to 2 teaspoons dried tarragon
4 tablespoons extra-virgin olive oil, for serving

1. Preheat the oven to 425°F (218°C). Line a baking sheet with parchment paper. 2. Place the salmon pieces, skin-side down, on a baking sheet. 3. In a small bowl, whisk together the mayonnaise, mustard, lemon zest and juice, tarragon, salt, and pepper. Top the salmon evenly with the sauce mixture. 4. Bake until slightly browned on top and slightly translucent in the center, 10 to 12 minutes, depending on the thickness of the salmon. Remove from the oven and leave on the baking sheet for 10 minutes. Drizzle each fillet with 1 tablespoon olive oil before serving.

Per Serving
Calories: 387 | Total Fat: 28g | Total Carbs: 4g | Net Carbs: 3g | Fiber: 1g | Protein: 29g | Sodium: 633mg

Greek Fish Pitas

Prep time: 10 minutes | Cook time: 15 minutes | Serves 4

1 pound (454 g) pollock, cut into 1-inch pieces
1 teaspoon salt
½ teaspoon dried thyme
¼ teaspoon cayenne
1 cup shredded lettuce
Nonfat plain Greek yogurt
¼ cup olive oil
½ teaspoon dried oregano
½ teaspoon garlic powder
4 whole wheat pitas
2 Roma tomatoes, diced
Lemon, quartered

1. Preheat the air fryer to 380°F (193°C). 2. In a medium bowl, combine the pollock with olive oil, salt, oregano, thyme, garlic powder, and cayenne. 3. Put the pollock into the air fryer basket and roast for 15 minutes. 4. Serve inside pitas with lettuce, tomato, and Greek yogurt with a lemon wedge on the side.

Per Serving
Calories: 368 | Total Fat: 16g | Saturated Fat: 2g | Protein: 21g | Total Carbohydrates: 38g | Fiber: 6g | Sugar: 2g | Cholesterol: 52mg

Italian Baccalà

Prep time: 2 to 3 hours | Cook time: 4 to 6 hours | Serves 4

1½ pounds (680 g) salt cod
½ onion, chopped
½ teaspoon red pepper flakes
Juice of ½ lemon
1 (15 ounces / 425-g) can no-salt-added diced tomatoes
2 garlic cloves, minced
¼ cup chopped fresh parsley, plus more for garnish

1. Wash the salt cod to remove any visible salt. Completely submerge the cod in a large bowl of water and let it soak for at least 2 to 3 hours. If you are soaking it for longer than 24 hours, change the water after 12 hours. 2. In a slow cooker, combine the tomatoes, onion, garlic, red pepper flakes, parsley, and lemon juice. Stir to mix well. Drain the cod and add it to the slow cooker, breaking it apart as necessary to make it fit. 3. Cover the cooker and cook for 4 to 6 hours on Low heat. 4. Garnish with the remaining fresh parsley for serving.

Per Serving
Calories: 211 | Total fat: 2g | Sodium: 179mg | Carbohydrates: 8g | Fiber: 2g | Sugar: 4g | Protein: 39g

Poached Salmon

Prep time: 10 minutes | Cook time: 5 minutes | Serves 4

1 lemon, sliced ¼ inch thick
½ teaspoon table salt
¼ teaspoon pepper
4 (6 ounces / 170 g) skinless salmon fillets, 1½ inches thick

1. Add ½ cup water to Instant Pot. Fold sheet of aluminum foil into 16 by 6-inch sling. Arrange lemon slices widthwise in 2 rows across center of sling. Sprinkle flesh side of salmon with salt and pepper, then arrange skinned side down on top of lemon slices. 2. Using sling, lower salmon into Instant Po; allow narrow edges of sling to rest along sides of insert. Lock lid in place and close pressure release valve. Select high pressure cook function and cook for 3 minutes. 3. Turn off Instant Pot and quick-release pressure. Carefully remove lid, allowing steam to escape away from you. Using sling, transfer salmon to large plate. Gently lift and tilt fillets with spatula to remove lemon slices. Serve.

Per Serving
Cal: 350 | Total Fat: 23g | Sat Fat: 5g | Chol: 95mg | Sodium: 390mg | Total Carbs: 0g, Fiber: 0g, Total Sugar: 0g | Added Sugar: 0g | Protein: 35g

Paprika-Spiced Fish

Prep time: 5 minutes | Cook time: 10 minutes | Serves 4

4 (5 ounces) sea bass fillets
1 tablespoon smoked paprika
Lemon wedges

½ teaspoon salt
3 tablespoons unsalted butter

1. Season the fish on both sides with the salt. Repeat with the paprika. 2. Preheat a skillet over high heat. Melt the butter. 3. Once the butter is melted, add the fish and cook for 4 minutes on each side. 4. Once the fish is done cooking, move to a serving dish and squeeze lemon over the top.

Per Serving
Calories: 257 | Protein: 34 | Total Carbohydrates: 1g | Sugars: 0g | Fiber: 1g | Total Fat: 13g | Saturated Fat: 6g | Cholesterol: 98mg | Sodium: 416mg

Monkfish with Sautéed Leeks, Fennel, and Tomatoes

Prep time: 20 minutes | Cook time: 35 minutes | Serves 4

1 to 1½ pounds (454 to 680 g) monkfish
1 teaspoon kosher salt, divided
2 tablespoons extra-virgin olive oil
½ onion, julienned
3 garlic cloves, minced
1 (14½ ounces / 411-g) can no-salt-added diced tomatoes
2 tablespoons fresh oregano, chopped

3 tablespoons lemon juice, divided
⅛ teaspoon freshly ground black pepper
1 leek, white and light green parts only, sliced in half lengthwise and thinly sliced
2 bupounds fennel, cored and thinly sliced, plus ¼ cup fronds for garnish
2 tablespoons fresh parsley, chopped
¼ teaspoon red pepper flakes

1. Place the fish in a medium baking dish and add 2 tablespoons of the lemon juice, ¼ teaspoon of the salt, and the black pepper. Place in the refrigerator. 2. Heat the olive oil in a large skillet or sauté pan over medium heat. Add the leek and onion and sauté until translucent, about 3 minutes. Add the garlic and sauté for 30 seconds. Add the fennel and sauté 4 to 5 minutes. Add the tomatoes and simmer for 2 to 3 minutes. 3. Stir in the parsley, oregano, red pepper flakes, the remaining ¾ teaspoon salt, and the remaining 1 tablespoon lemon juice. Place the fish on top of the leek mixture, cover, and simmer for 20 to 25 minutes, turning over halfway through, until the fish is opaque and pulls apart easily. Garnish with the fennel fronds.

Per Serving
Calories: 220 | Fat: 9g | Protein: 22g | Carbs: 11g | Sugars: 6g | Fiber: 3g | Sodium: 345mg | Cholesterol: 35mg

Shrimp Foil Packets

Prep time: 15 minutes | Cook time: 4 to 6 hours | Serves 4

1½ pounds (680 g) whole raw medium shrimp, peeled, deveined, and divided into 4 (6 ounces / 170 g) portions
4 teaspoons balsamic vinegar, divided
1 red onion, cut into chunks
4 Roma tomatoes, chopped
Juice of 1 lemon

Sea salt
Freshly ground black pepper
2 teaspoons extra-virgin olive oil, divided
4 garlic cloves, minced
1 large zucchini, sliced
4 teaspoons dried oregano, divided

1. Place a large sheet of aluminum foil on a work surface. Lay one-quarter of the shrimp in the center of the foil and season it with salt and pepper. Drizzle with ½ teaspoon of olive oil and 1 teaspoon of vinegar. 2. Top the shrimp with one-quarter each of the garlic, onion, and zucchini, plus 1 tomato and 1 teaspoon of oregano. Place a second sheet of foil on top of the ingredients. Fold the corners over to seal the packet. 3. Repeat to make 3 more foil packets. Place the packets in a slow cooker in a single layer, or stack them if needed. 4. Cover the cooker and cook for 4 to 6 hours on Low heat. 5. Be careful when serving: Very hot steam will release when you open the foil packets. Drizzle each opened packet with lemon juice for serving.

Per Serving
Calories: 210 | Total fat: 5g | Sodium: 187mg | Carbohydrates: 17g | Fiber: 3g | Sugar: 9g | Protein: 30g

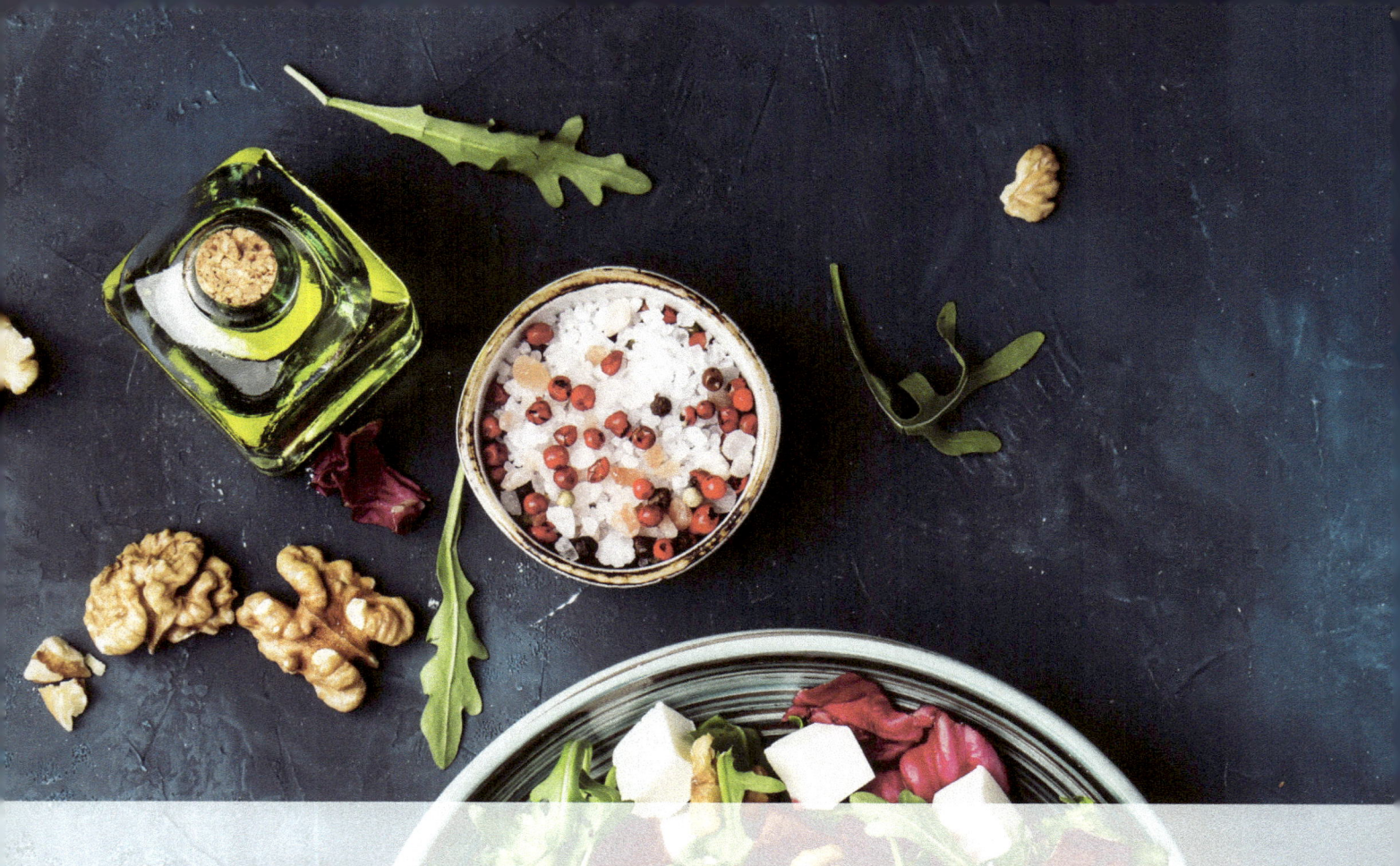

Chapter 7   Meatless Mains

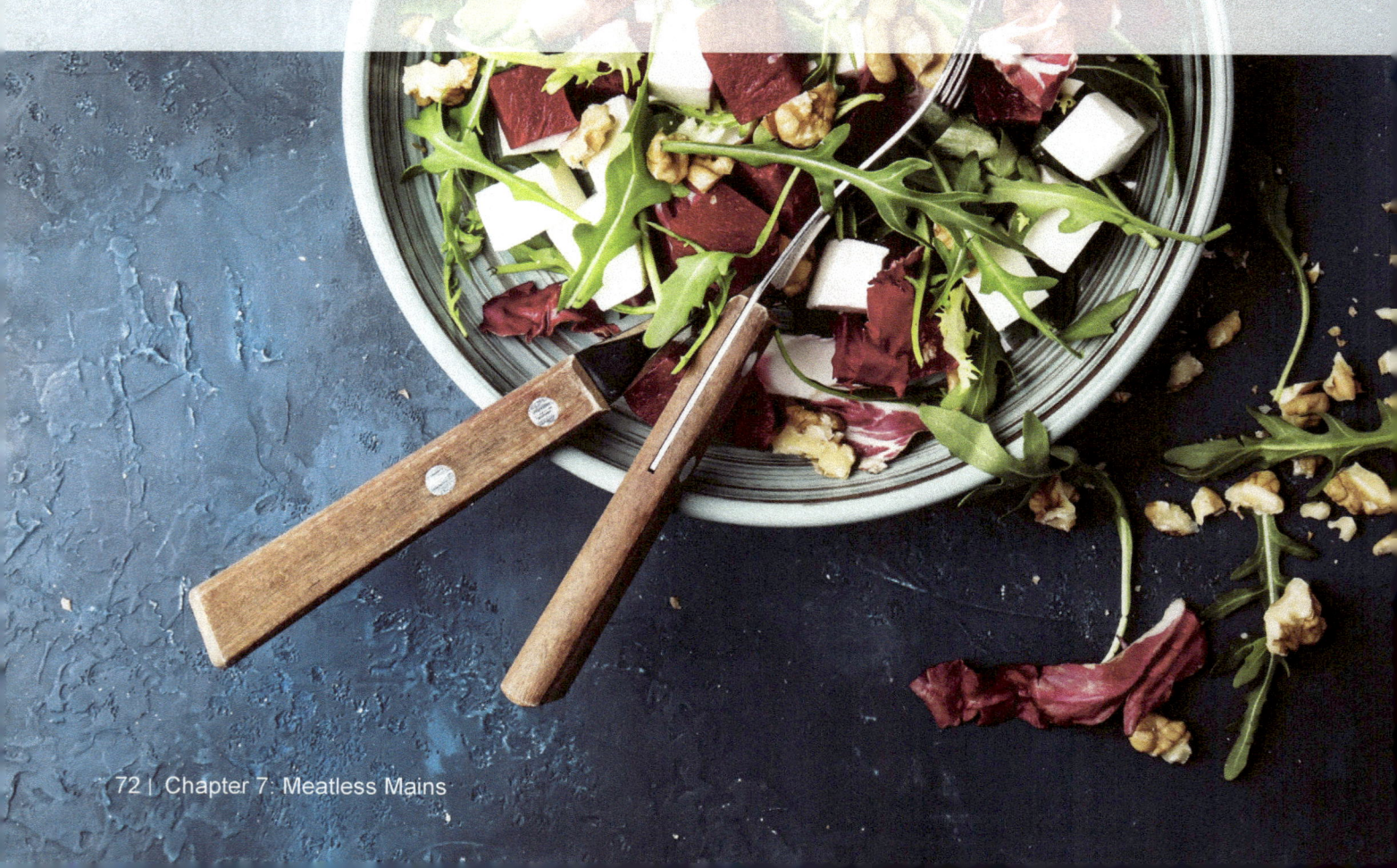

111 **Sweet Veggie-Stuffed Peppers** 74

112 **Moussaka** 74

113 **Vegetable-Stuffed Grape Leaves** 75

114 **Grilled Eggplant Rolls** 75

115 **Cheesy Spinach Pies** 76

116 **Moroccan-Style Couscous** 76

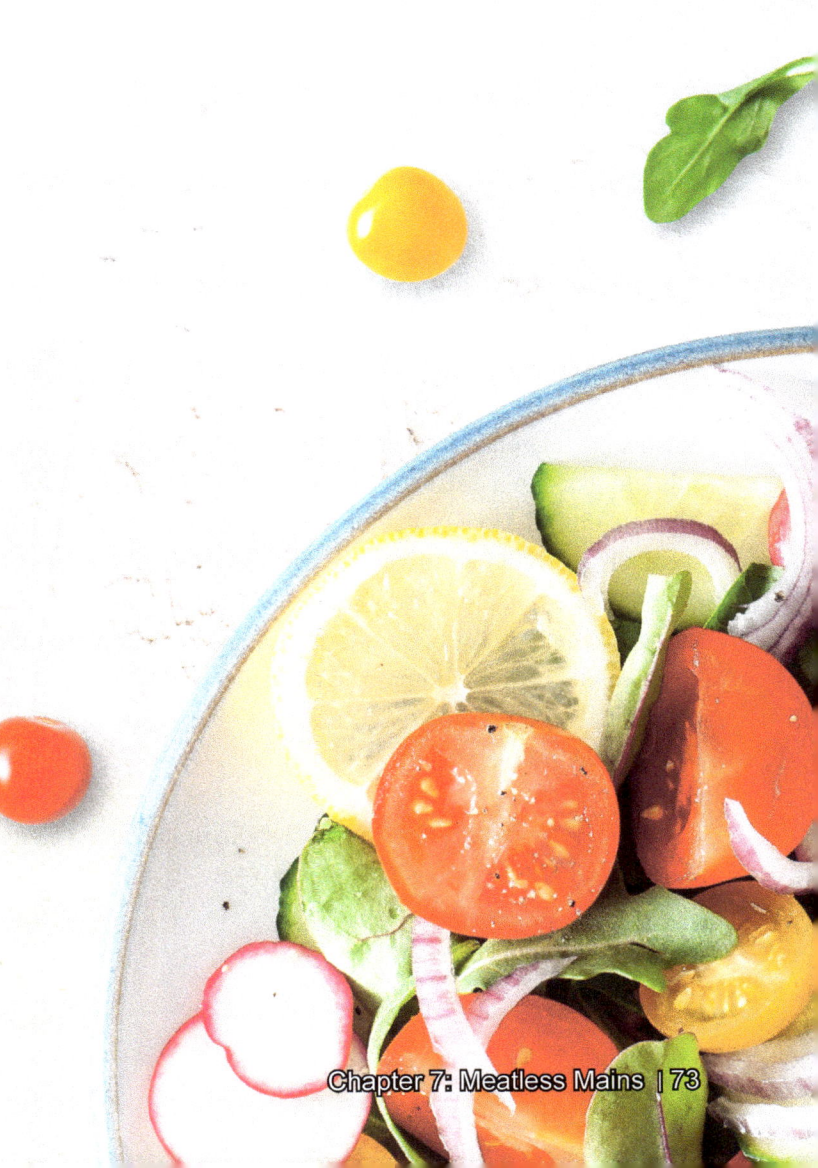

Sweet Veggie-Stuffed Peppers

Prep time: 20 minutes | Cook time: 30 minutes | Serves 4

6 large bell peppers, different colors
1 large onion, chopped
1 carrot, chopped
3 cups cooked rice
1½ teaspoons salt
3 tablespoons extra-virgin olive oil
3 cloves garlic, minced
1 (16 ounces / 454 g) can garbanzo beans, rinsed and drained
½ teaspoon freshly ground black pepper

1. Preheat the oven to 350°F (177°C). 2. Make sure to choose peppers that can stand upright. Cut off the pepper cap and remove the seeds, reserving the cap for later. Stand the peppers in a baking dish. 3. In a large skillet over medium heat, cook the olive oil, onion, garlic, and carrots for 3 minutes. 4. Stir in the garbanzo beans. Cook for another 3 minutes. 5. Remove the pan from the heat and spoon the cooked ingredients to a large bowl. 6. Add the rice, salt, and pepper; toss to combine. 7. Stuff each pepper to the top and then put the pepper caps back on. 8. Cover the baking dish with aluminum foil and bake for 25 minutes. 9. Remove the foil and bake for another 5 minutes. 10. Serve warm.

Per Serving
Calories: 301 | Protein: 8g | Total Carbohydrates: 50g | Sugars: 8g | Fiber: 8g | Total Fat: 9g | Saturated Fat: 1g | Cholesterol: 0mg | Sodium: 597mg

Moussaka

Prep time: 55 minutes | Cook time: 40 minutes | Serves 6

2 large eggplants
Olive oil spray, or olive oil for brushing
2 large onions, sliced
2 (15 ounces / 425-g) cans diced tomatoes
1 teaspoon dried oregano
½ teaspoon freshly ground black pepper
2 teaspoons salt, divided
¼ cup extra-virgin olive oil
10 cloves garlic, sliced
1 (16 ounces / 454 g) can garbanzo beans, rinsed and drained

1. Slice the eggplant horizontally into ¼-inch-thick round disks. Sprinkle the eggplant slices with 1 teaspoon of salt and place in a colander for 30 minutes. This will draw out the excess water from the eggplant. 2. Preheat the oven to 450°F (235°C). Pat the slices of eggplant dry with a paper towel and spray each side with an olive oil spray or lightly brush each side with olive oil. 3. Arrange the eggplant in a single layer on a baking sheet. Put in the oven and bake for 10 minutes. Then, using a spatula, flip the slices over and bake for another 10 minutes. 4. In a large skillet add the olive oil, onions, garlic, and remaining 1 teaspoon of salt. Cook for 3 to 5 minutes stirring occasionally. Add the tomatoes, garbanzo beans, oregano, and black pepper. Simmer for 10 to 12 minutes, stirring occasionally. 5. Using a deep casserole dish, begin to layer, starting with eggplant, then the sauce. Repeat until all ingredients have been used. Bake in the oven for 20 minutes. 6. Remove from the oven and serve warm.

Per Serving
Calories: 262 | Protein: 8g | Total Carbohydrates: 35g | Sugars: 14g | Fiber: 11g | Total Fat: 11g | Saturated Fat: 1g | Cholesterol: 0mg | Sodium: 1,043mg

Vegetable-Stuffed Grape Leaves

Prep time: 50 minutes | Cook time: 45 minutes | Serves 6 to 8

- 2 cups white rice, rinsed
- 1 large onion, finely chopped
- 1 cup fresh Italian parsley, finely chopped
- 2½ teaspoons salt
- 1 (16 ounces / 454 g) jar grape leaves
- ½ cup extra-virgin olive oil
- 2 large tomatoes, finely diced
- 1 green onion, finely chopped
- 3 cloves garlic, minced
- ½ teaspoon freshly ground black pepper
- 1 cup lemon juice
- 4 to 6 cups water

1. In a large bowl, combine the rice, tomatoes, onion, green onion, parsley, garlic, salt, and black pepper. 2. Drain and rinse the grape leaves. 3. Prepare a large pot by placing a layer of grape leaves on the bottom. Lay each leaf flat and trim off any stems. 4. Place 2 tablespoons of the rice mixture at the base of each leaf. Fold over the sides, then roll as tight as possible. Place the rolled grape leaves in the pot, lining up each rolled grape leaf. Continue to layer in the rolled grape leaves. 5. Gently pour the lemon juice and olive oil over the grape leaves, and add enough water to just cover the grape leaves by 1 inch. 6. Lay a heavy plate that is smaller than the opening of the pot upside down over the grape leaves. Cover the pot and cook the leaves over medium-low heat for 45 minutes. Let stand for 20 minutes before serving. 7. Serve warm or cold.

Per Serving

Calories: 532 | Protein: 12g | Total Carbohydrates: 80g | Sugars: 9g | Fiber: 15g | Total Fat: 21g | Saturated Fat: 3g | Cholesterol: 0mg | Sodium: 995mg

Grilled Eggplant Rolls

Prep time: 30 minutes | Cook time: 10 minutes | Serves 4 to 6

- 2 large eggplants
- 4 ounces (113 g) goat cheese
- ¼ cup fresh basil, finely chopped
- Olive oil spray
- 1 teaspoon salt
- 1 cup ricotta
- ½ teaspoon freshly ground black pepper

1. Trim off the tops of the eggplants and cut the eggplants lengthwise into ¼-inch-thick slices. Sprinkle the slices with the salt and place the eggplant in a colander for 15 to 20 minutes. The salt will draw out excess water from the eggplant. 2. In a large bowl, combine the goat cheese, ricotta, basil, and pepper. 3. Preheat a grill, grill pan, or lightly oiled skillet on medium heat. Pat the eggplant slices dry with a paper towel and lightly spray with olive oil spray. Place the eggplant on the grill, grill pan, or skillet and cook for 3 minutes on each side. 4. Remove the eggplant from the heat and let cool for 5 minutes. 5. To roll, lay one eggplant slice flat, place a tablespoon of the cheese mixture at the base of the slice, and roll up. Serve immediately or chill until serving.

Per Serving

Calories: 255 | Protein: 15g | Total Carbohydrates: 19g | Sugars: 10g | Fiber: 7g | Total Fat: 15g | Saturated Fat: 9g | Cholesterol: 44mg | Sodium: 746mg

Cheesy Spinach Pies

Prep time: 20 minutes | Cook time: 40 minutes | Serves 6 to 8

- 2 tablespoons extra-virgin olive oil
- 2 cloves garlic, minced
- 1 cup feta cheese
- Puff pastry sheets
- 1 large onion, chopped
- 3 (1-pound) bags of baby spinach, washed
- 1 large egg, beaten

1. Preheat the oven to 375°F (191°C). 2. In a large skillet over medium heat, cook the olive oil, onion, and garlic for 3 minutes. 3. Add the spinach to the skillet one bag at a time, letting it wilt in between each bag. Toss using tongs. Cook for 4 minutes. Once the spinach is cooked, drain any excess liquid from the pan. 4. In a large bowl, combine the feta cheese, egg, and cooked spinach. 5. Lay the puff pastry flat on a counter. Cut the pastry into 3-inch squares. 6. Place a tablespoon of the spinach mixture in the center of a puff-pastry square. Fold over one corner of the square to the diagonal corner, forming a triangle. Crimp the edges of the pie by pressing down with the tines of a fork to seal them together. Repeat until all squares are filled. 7. Place the pies on a parchment-lined baking sheet and bake for 25 to 30 minutes or until golden brown. Serve warm or at room temperature.

Per Serving

Calories: 503 | Protein: 16g | Total Carbohydrates: 38g | Sugars: 4g | Fiber: 6g | Total Fat: 32g | Saturated Fat: 10g | Cholesterol: 53mg | Sodium: 843mg

Moroccan-Style Couscous

Prep timePrep Time: 10 minutes | Cook Time: 5 minutes | Serves 2

- 1 tablespoon olive oil
- ¼ teaspoon garlic powder
- ¼ teaspoon cinnamon
- 2 tablespoons raisins
- 2 teaspoons minced fresh parsley
- ¾ cup couscous
- ¼ teaspoon salt
- 1 cup water
- 2 tablespoons minced dried apricots

1. Heat the olive oil in a saucepan over medium-high heat. Add the couscous, garlic powder, salt, and cinnamon. Stir for 1 minute to toast the couscous and spices. 2. Add the water, raisins, and apricots and bring the mixture to a boil. 3. Cover the pot and turn off the heat. Let the couscous sit for 4 to 5 minutes and then fluff it with a fork. Add parsley and season with additional salt or spices as needed.

Per Serving

Calories: 338 | Total fat: 8g | Total carbs: 59g | Fiber: 4g | Sugar: 6g | Protein: 9g | Sodium: 299mg | Cholesterol: 0mg

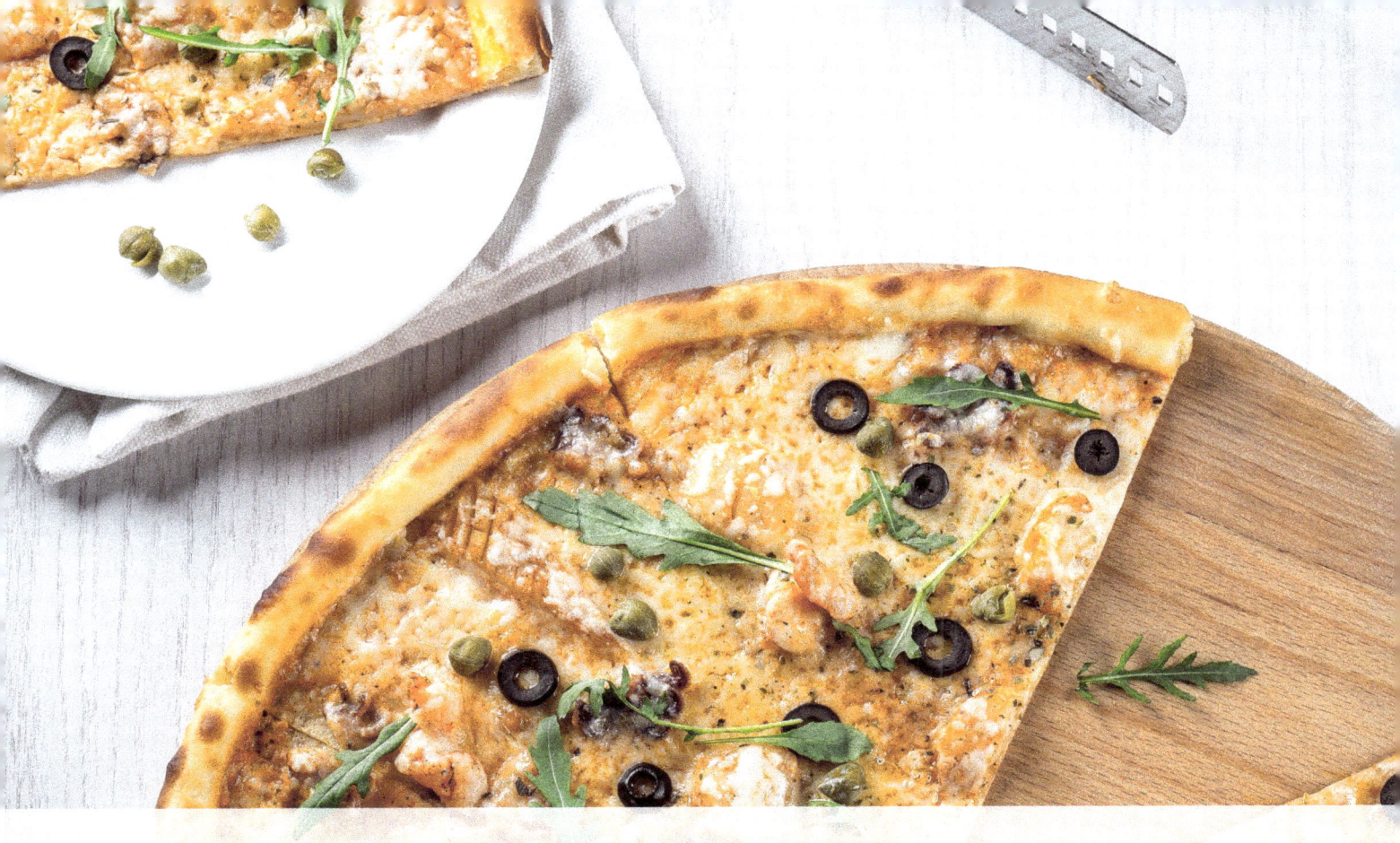

Chapter 8   Pizzas, Wraps, and Sandwiches

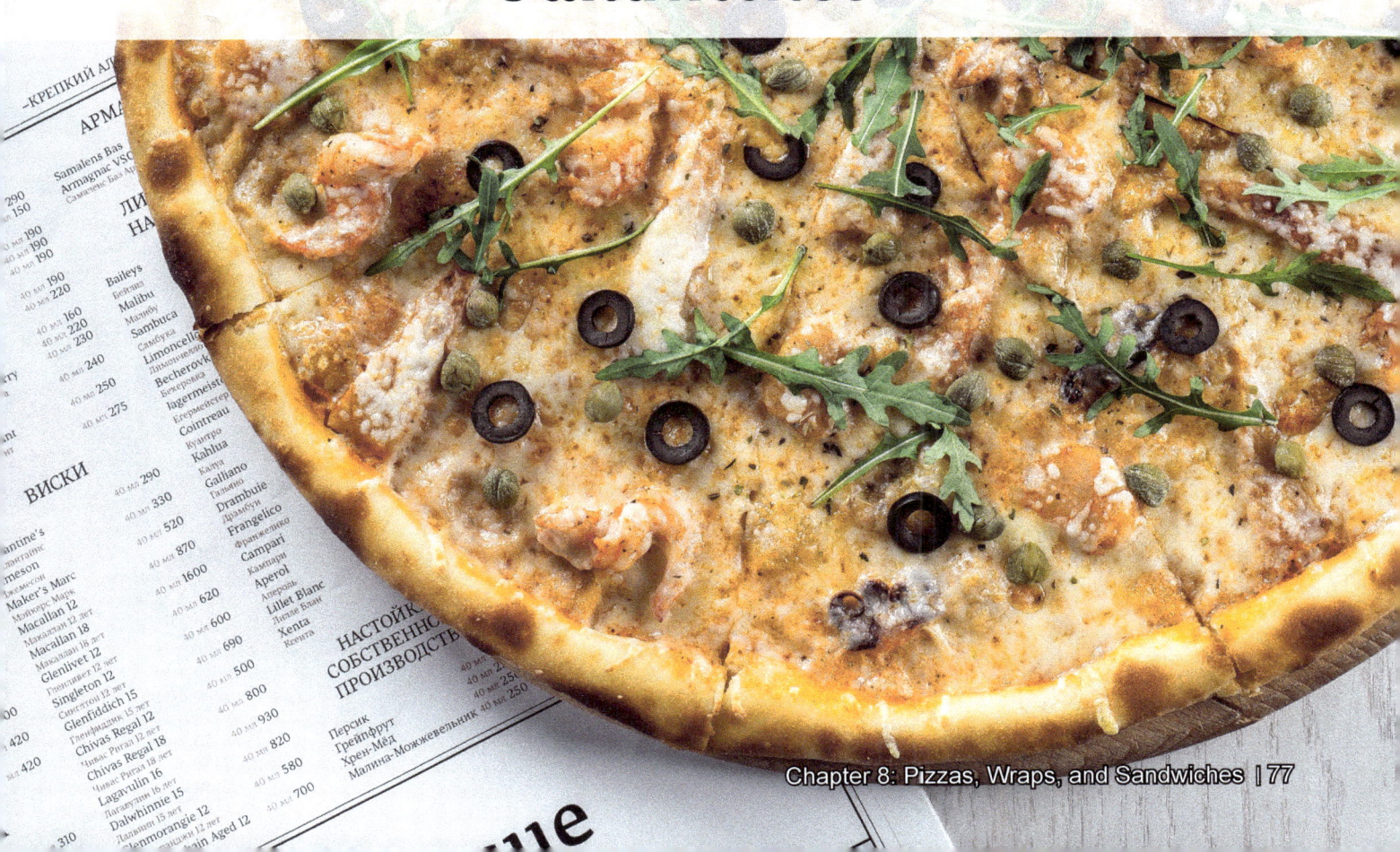

117 **Chicken and Goat Cheese Pizza** 79

118 **Roasted Vegetable Bocadillo with Romesco Sauce** 79

119 **White Pizza with Prosciutto and Arugula** 79

120 **Turkey and Provolone Panini with Roasted Peppers and Onions** 80

121 **Bocadillo with Herbed Tuna and Piquillo Peppers** 80

122 **Sautéed Mushroom, Onion, and Pecorino Romano Panini** 81

123 **Moroccan Lamb Wrap with Harissa** 81

124 **Classic Margherita Pizza** 82

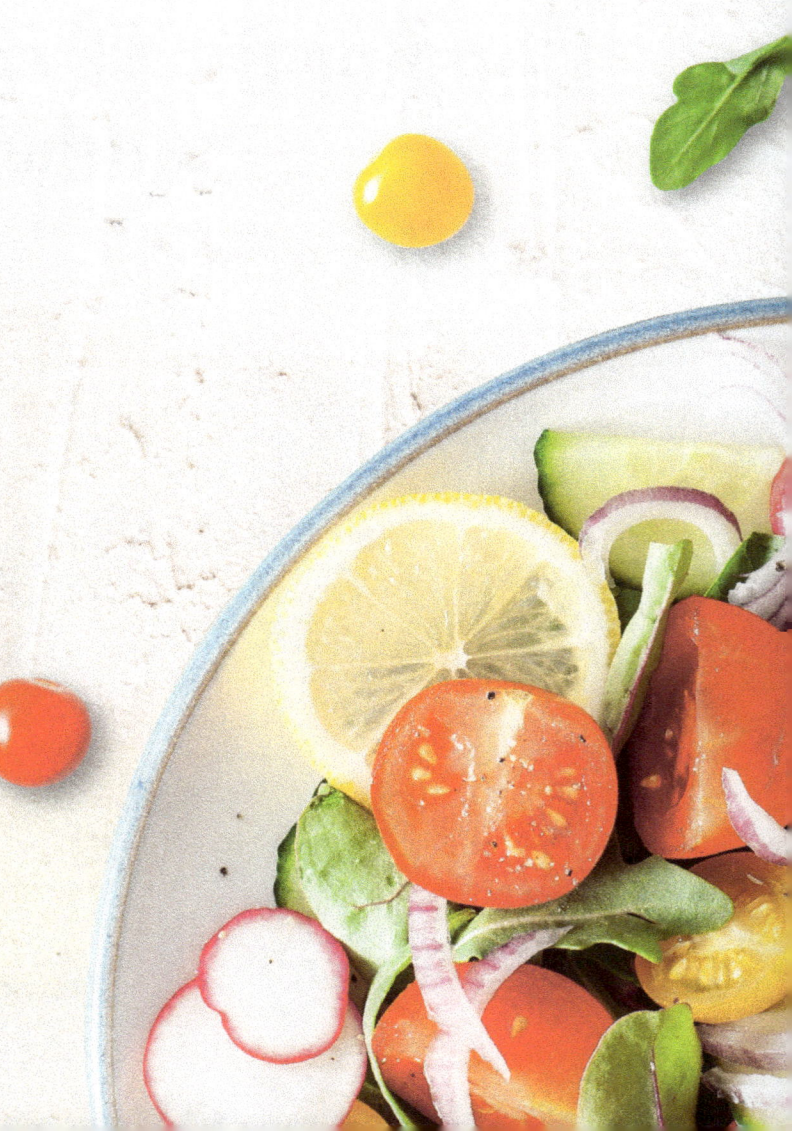

Chicken and Goat Cheese Pizza

Prep time: 10 minutes | Cook time: 10 minutes | Serves 4

- All-purpose flour, for dusting
- 2 tablespoons olive oil
- 3 ounces goat cheese, crumbled
- Freshly ground black pepper
- 1 pound (454 g) premade pizza dough
- 1 cup shredded cooked chicken
- Sea salt

1. Preheat the oven to 475°F (246°C). 2. On a floured surface, roll out the dough to a 12-inch round and place it on a lightly floured pizza pan or baking sheet. Drizzle the dough with the olive oil and spread it out evenly. Top the dough with the chicken and goat cheese. 3. Bake the pizza for 8 to 10 minutes, until the crust is cooked through and golden. 4. Season with salt and pepper and serve.

Per Serving
Calories: 593 | Total fat: 21g | Total carbs: 70g | Sugar: 8g | Protein: 31g | Fiber: 4g | Sodium: 924mg

Roasted Vegetable Bocadillo with Romesco Sauce

Prep time: 10 minutes | Cook time: 20 minutes | Serves 4

- 2 small yellow squash, sliced lengthwise
- 1 medium red onion, thinly sliced
- 2 tablespoons olive oil
- ½ teaspoon freshly ground black pepper, divided
- 2 tablespoons blanched almonds
- 1 small clove garlic
- 4 ounces (113 g) goat cheese, at room temperature
- 2 small zucchini, sliced lengthwise
- 4 large button mushrooms, sliced
- 1 teaspoon salt, divided
- 2 roasted red peppers from a jar, drained
- 1 tablespoon sherry vinegar
- 4 crusty multigrain rolls
- 1 tablespoon chopped fresh basil

1. Preheat the oven to 400°F (204°C). 2. In a medium bowl, toss the yellow squash, zucchini, onion, and mushrooms with the olive oil, ½ teaspoon salt, and ¼ teaspoon pepper. Spread on a large baking sheet. Roast the vegetables in the oven for about 20 minutes, until softened. 3. Meanwhile, in a food processor, combine the roasted peppers, almonds, vinegar, garlic, the remaining ½ teaspoon salt, and the remaining ¼ teaspoon pepper and process until smooth. 4. Split the rolls and spread ¼ of the goat cheese on the bottom of each. Place the roasted vegetables on top of the cheese, dividing equally. Top with chopped basil. Spread the top halves of the rolls with the roasted red pepper sauce and serve immediately.

Per Serving
Calories: 394 | Total Fat: 20g | Saturated Fat: 8g | Carbs: 37g | Protein: 21g | Sodium: 954mg | Fiber: 8g

White Pizza with Prosciutto and Arugula

Prep time: 10 minutes | Cook time: 15 minutes | Serves 4

- 1 pound (454 g) prepared pizza dough
- 1 tablespoon garlic, minced
- 3 ounces prosciutto, thinly sliced
- ½ teaspoon freshly ground black pepper
- ½ cup ricotta cheese
- 1 cup grated mozzarella cheese
- ½ cup fresh arugula

1. Preheat the oven to 450°F (235°C). Roll out the pizza dough on a floured surface. 2. Put the pizza dough on a parchment-lined baking sheet or pizza sheet. Put the dough in the oven and bake for 8 minutes. 3. In a small bowl, mix together the ricotta, garlic, and mozzarella. 4. Remove the pizza dough from the oven and spread the cheese mixture over the top. Bake for another 5 to 6 minutes. 5. Top the pizza with prosciutto, arugula, and peppe; serve warm.

Per Serving
Calories: 435 | Protein: 20g | Total Carbohydrates: 51g | Sugars: 0g | Fiber: 4g | Total Fat: 17g | Saturated Fat: 8g | Cholesterol: 53mg | Sodium: 1,630mg

Turkey and Provolone Panini with Roasted Peppers and Onions

Prep time: 15 minutes | Cook time: 1 hour 5 minutes | Serves 4

For the peppers and onions

2 red bell pepper, seeded and quartered
2 tablespoons olive oil
½ teaspoon freshly ground black pepper
2 red onions, peeled and quartered
½ teaspoon salt

For the panini

2 tablespoons olive oil
8 ounces (227 g) thinly sliced provolone cheese
8 slices whole-wheat bread
8 ounces (227 g) sliced roasted turkey or chicken breast

1. Preheat the oven to 375°F (191°C). 2. To roast the peppers and onions, toss them together with the olive oil, salt, and pepper on a large, rimmed baking sheet. Spread them out in a single layer and then bake in the preheated oven for 45 to 60 minutes, turning occasionally, until they are tender and beginning to brown. Remove the peppers and onions from the oven and let them cool for a few minutes until they are cool enough to handle. Skin the peppers and thinly slice them. Thinly slice the onions. 3. Preheat a skillet or grill pan over medium-high heat. 4. To make the panini, brush one side of each of the 8 slices of bread with olive oil. Place 4 of the bread slices, oiled side down, on your work surface. Top each with ¼ of the cheese and ¼ of the turkey, and top with some of the roasted peppers and onions. Place the remaining 4 bread slices on top of the sandwiches, oiled side up. 5. Place the sandwiches in the skillet or grill pan (you may have to cook them in two batches), cover the pan, and cook until the bottoms have golden brown grill marks and the cheese is beginning to melt, about 2 minutes. Turn the sandwiches over and cook, covered, until the second side is golden brown and the cheese is melted, another 2 minutes or so. Cut each sandwich in half and serve immediately.

Per Serving

Calories: 562 | Total Fat: 33g | Saturated Fat: 12g | Carbs: 38g | Protein: 31g | Sodium: 1,737mg | Fiber: 6.5g

Bocadillo with Herbed Tuna and Piquillo Peppers

Prep time: 5 minutes | Cook time: 20 minutes | Serves 4

2 tablespoons olive oil, plus more for brushing
2 leeks, white and tender green parts only, finely chopped
½ teaspoon salt
3 tablespoons sherry vinegar
2 (8 ounces / 227 g)) jars Spanish tuna in olive oil
1 ripe tomato, grated on the large holes of a box grater
1 medium onion, finely chopped
1 teaspoon chopped thyme
½ teaspoon dried marjoram
¼ teaspoon freshly ground black pepper
1 carrot, finely diced
4 crusty whole-wheat sandwich rolls, split
4 piquillo peppers, cut into thin strips

1. Heat 2 tablespoons olive oil in a medium skillet over medium heat. Add the onion, leeks, thyme, marjoram, salt, and pepper. Stir frequently until the onions are softened, about 10 minutes. Stir in the vinegar and carrot and cook until the liquid has evaporated, 5 minutes. Transfer the mixture to a bowl and let cool to room temperature or refrigerate for 15 minutes or so. 2. In a medium bowl, combine the tuna, along with its oil, with the onion mixture, breaking the tuna chunks up with a fork. 3. Brush the rolls lightly with oil and toast under the broiler until lightly browned, about 2 minutes. Spoon the tomato pulp onto the bottom half of each roll, dividing equally and spreading it with the back of the spoon. Divide the tuna mixture among the rolls and top with the piquillo pepper slices. Serve immediately.

Per Serving

Calories: 412 | Total Fat: 23g | Saturated Fat: 3g | Carbs: 26g | Protein: 31g | Sodium: 948mg | Fiber: 3g

Sautéed Mushroom, Onion, and Pecorino Romano Panini

Prep time: 10 minutes | Cook time: 20 minutes | Serves 4

3 tablespoons olive oil, divided

10 ounces button or cremini mushrooms, sliced

¼ teaspoon freshly ground black pepper

4 ounces (113 g) freshly grated Pecorino Romano

1 small onion, diced

½ teaspoon salt

4 crusty Italian sandwich rolls

1. Heat 1 tablespoon of the olive oil in a skillet over medium-high heat. Add the onion and cook, stirring, until it begins to soften, about 3 minutes. Add the mushrooms, season with salt and pepper, and cook, stirring, until they soften and the liquid they release evaporates, about 7 minutes. 2. To make the panini, heat a skillet or grill pan over high heat and brush with 1 tablespoon olive oil. Brush the inside of the rolls with the remaining 1 tablespoon olive oil. Divide the mushroom mixture evenly among the rolls and top each with ¼ of the grated cheese. 3. Place the sandwiches in the hot pan and place another heavy pan, such as a cast-iron skillet, on top to weigh them down. Cook for about 3 to 4 minutes, until crisp and golden on the bottom, and then flip over and repeat on the second side, cooking for an additional 3 to 4 minutes until golden and crisp. Slice each sandwich in half and serve hot.

Per Serving

Calories: 468 | Total Fat: 21g | Saturated Fat: 9g | Carbs: 52g | Protein: 19g | Sodium: 1,333mg | Fiber: 3g

Moroccan Lamb Wrap with Harissa

Prep time: 10 minutes | Cook time: 10 minutes | Serves 4

1 clove garlic, minced

2 teaspoons chopped fresh thyme

1 lamb leg steak, about 12 ounces

1 medium eggplant, sliced ½-inch thick

1 medium zucchini, sliced lengthwise into 4 slices

6 to 8 Kalamata olives, sliced

2 to 4 tablespoons harissa

2 teaspoons ground cumin

¼ cup olive oil, divided

4 (8-inch) pocketless pita rounds or naan, preferably whole-wheat

1 bell pepper (any color), roasted and skinned

Juice of 1 lemon

2 cups arugula

1. In a large bowl, combine the garlic, cumin, thyme, and 1 tablespoon of the olive oil. Add the lamb, turn to coat, cover, refrigerate, and marinate for at least an hour. 2. Preheat the oven to 400°F (204°C). 3. Heat a grill or grill pan to high heat. Remove the lamb from the marinade and grill for about 4 minutes per side, until medium-rare. Transfer to a plate and let rest for about 10 minutes before slicing thinly across the grain. 4. While the meat is resting, wrap the bread rounds in aluminum foil and heat in the oven for about 10 minutes. 5. Meanwhile, brush the eggplant and zucchini slices with the remaining olive oil and grill until tender, about 3 minutes. Dice them and the bell pepper. Toss in a large bowl with the olives and lemon juice. 6. Spread some of the harissa onto each warm flatbread round and top each evenly with roasted vegetables, a few slices of lamb, and a handful of the arugula. 7. Roll up the wraps, cut each in half crosswise, and serve immediately.

Per Serving

Calories: 553 | Total Fat: 24g | Saturated Fat: 5g | Carbs: 53g | Protein: 33g | Sodium: 531mg | Fiber: 11g

Classic Margherita Pizza

Prep time: 10 minutes | Cook time: 10 minutes | Serves 4

All-purpose flour, for dusting
1 (15 ounces / 425-g) can crushed San Marzano tomatoes, with their juices
Pinch sea salt, plus more as needed
10 slices mozzarella cheese
1 pound (454 g) premade pizza dough
2 garlic cloves
1 teaspoon Italian seasoning
1½ teaspoons olive oil, for drizzling
12 to 15 fresh basil leaves

1. Preheat the oven to 475°F (246°C). 2. On a floured surface, roll out the dough to a 12-inch round and place it on a lightly floured pizza pan or baking sheet. 3. In a food processor, combine the tomatoes with their juices, garlic, Italian seasoning, and salt and process until smooth. Taste and adjust the seasoning. 4. Drizzle the olive oil over the pizza dough, then spoon the pizza sauce over the dough and spread it out evenly with the back of the spoon, leaving a 1-inch border. Evenly distribute the mozzarella over the pizza. 5. Bake until the crust is cooked through and golden, 8 to 10 minutes. Remove from the oven and let sit for 1 to 2 minutes. Top with the basil right before serving.

Per Serving
Calories: 540 | Total fat: 21g | Total carbs: 62g | Sugar: 11g | Protein: 27g | Fiber: 5g | Sodium: 1,094mg

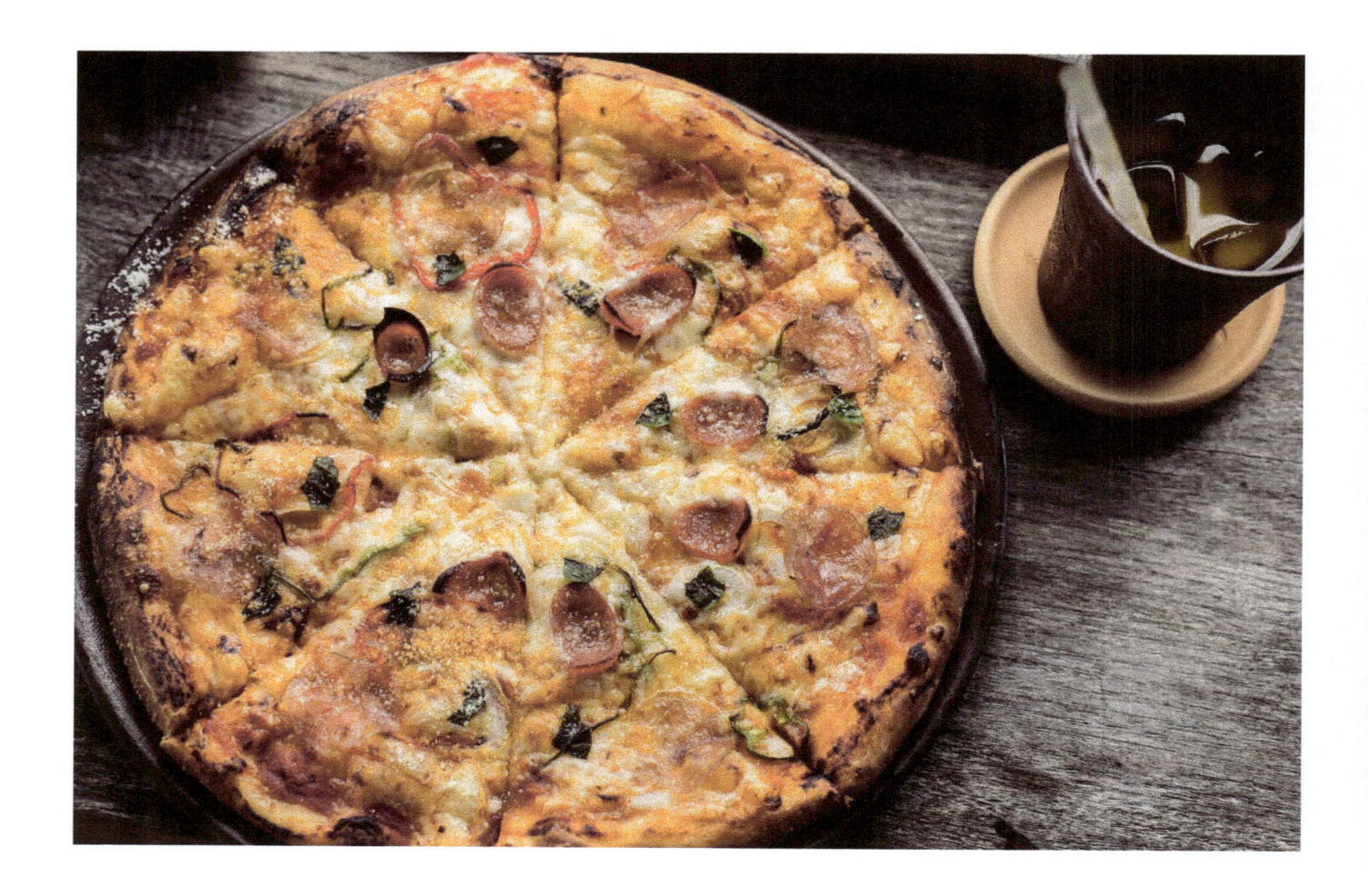

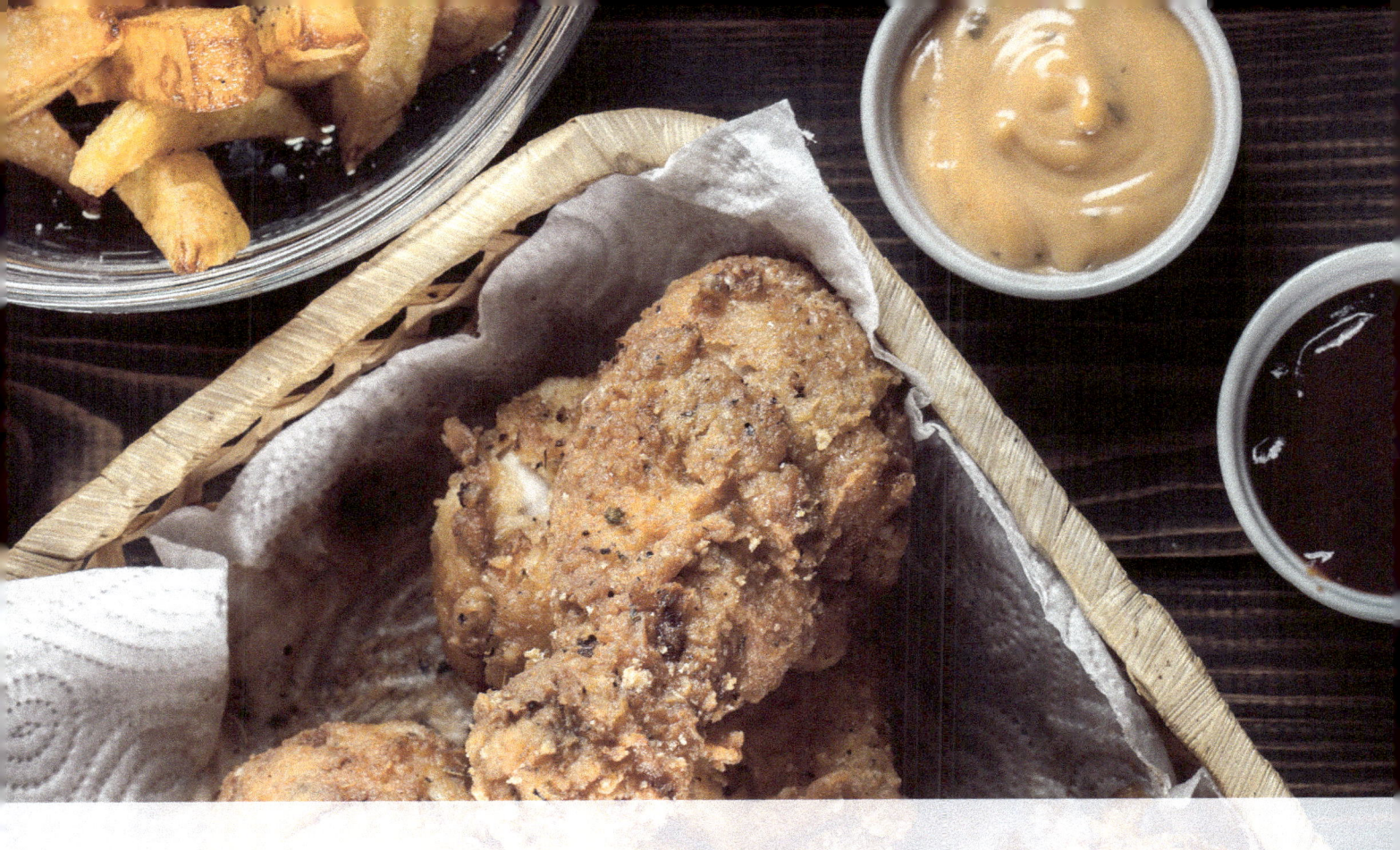

Chapter 9 Poultry

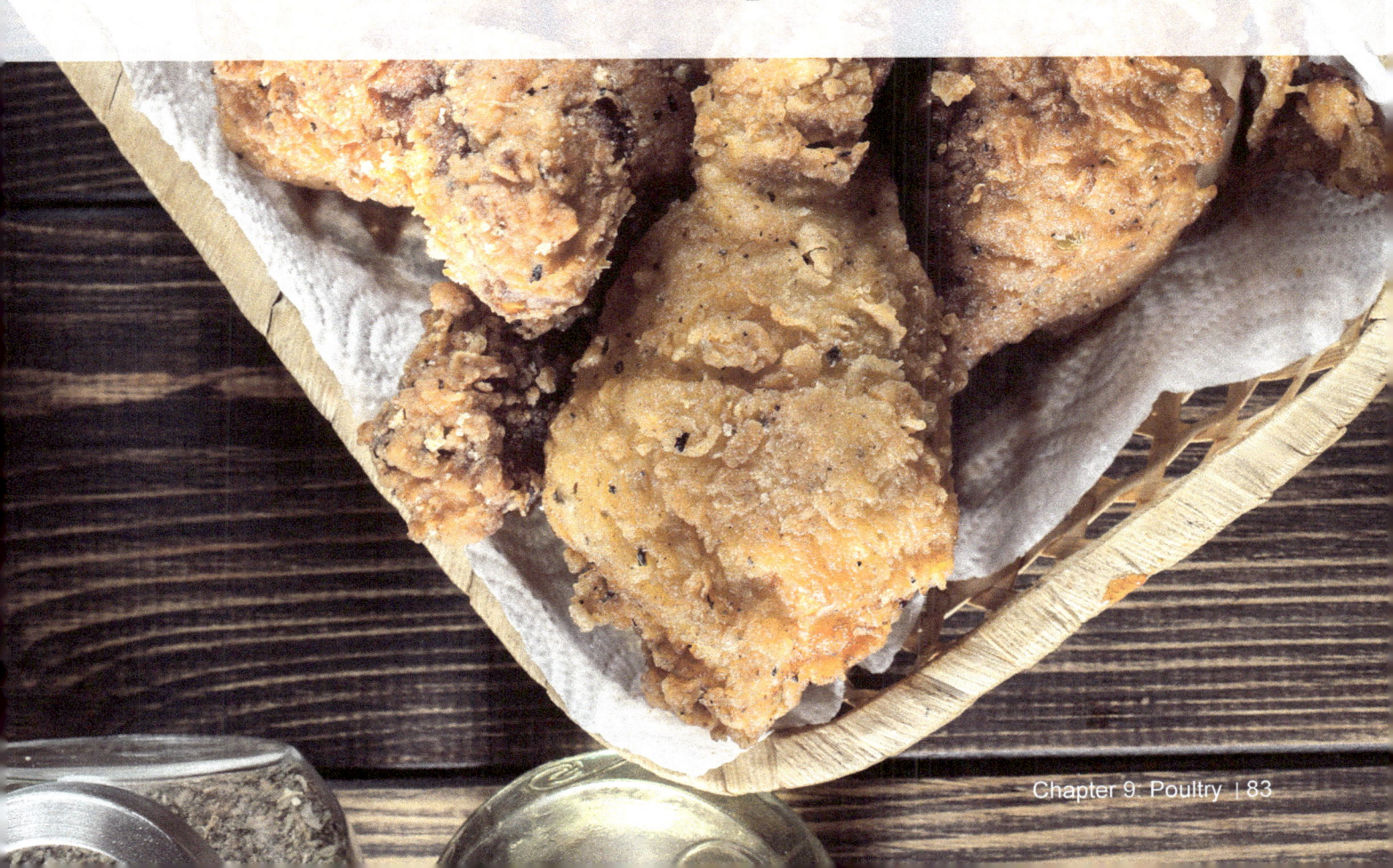

125 **Chicken Piccata with Mushrooms** 85

126 **Chicken Cutlets with Greek Salsa** 85

127 **Mediterranean Roasted Turkey Breast** 86

128 **Moroccan-Spiced Chicken Thighs with Saffron Basmati Rice** 86

129 **Chicken with Olives and Capers** 87

130 **Bomba Chicken with Chickpeas** 87

131 **Chicken Avgolemono** 87

132 **Kale, Chickpea, and Chicken Stew** 88

133 **Chicken with Lemon Asparagus** 88

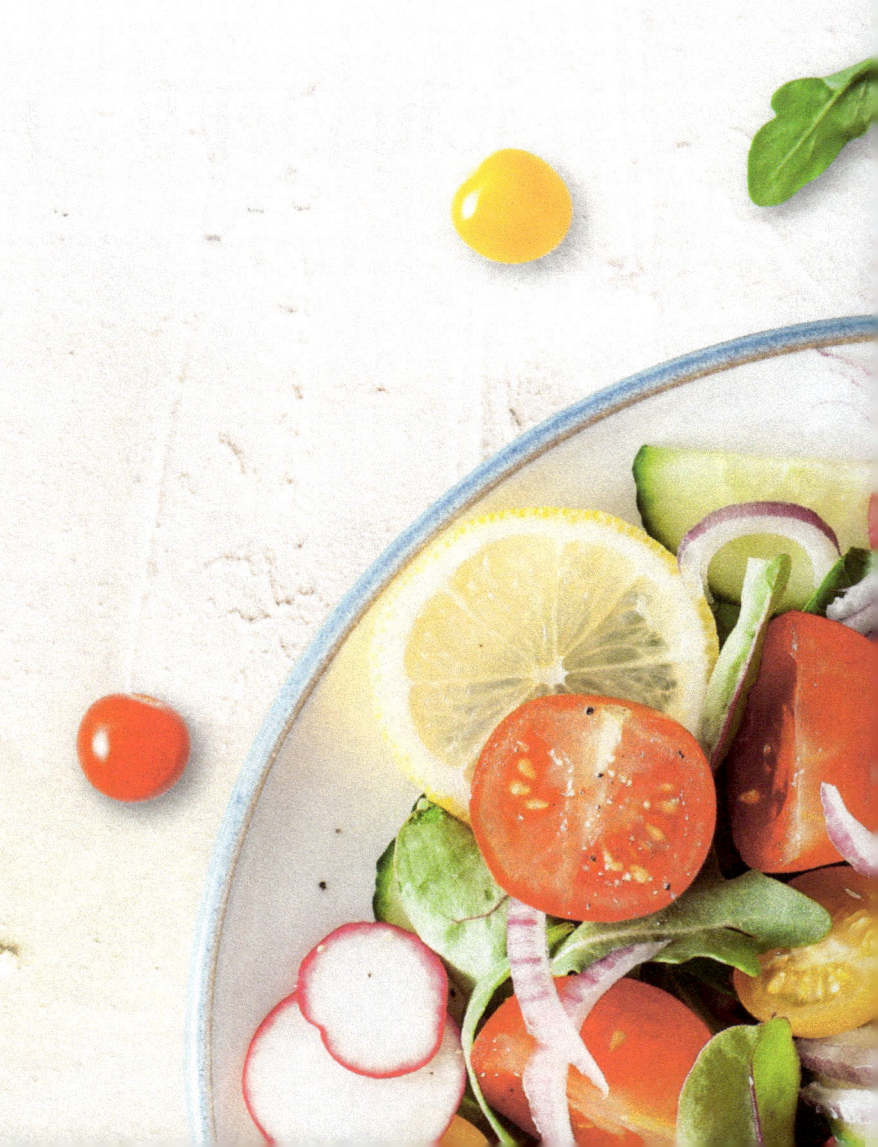

Chicken Piccata with Mushrooms

Prep time: 25 minutes | Cook time: 25 minutes | Serves 4

- 1 pound (454 g) thinly sliced chicken breasts
- ½ teaspoon freshly ground black pepper
- 2 tablespoons almond flour
- 4 tablespoons butter, divided
- ½ cup dry white wine or chicken stock
- ¼ cup roughly chopped capers
- ¼ cup chopped fresh flat-leaf Italian parsley, for garnish
- 1½ teaspoons salt, divided
- ¼ cup ground flaxseed
- 8 tablespoons extra-virgin olive oil, divided
- 2 cups sliced mushrooms
- ¼ cup freshly squeezed lemon juice
- Zucchini noodles, for serving

1. Season the chicken with 1 teaspoon salt and the pepper. On a plate, combine the ground flaxseed and almond flour and dredge each chicken breast in the mixture. Set aside. 2. In a large skillet, heat 4 tablespoons olive oil and 1 tablespoon butter over medium-high heat. Working in batches if necessary, brown the chicken, 3 to 4 minutes per side. Remove from the skillet and keep warm. 3. Add the remaining 4 tablespoons olive oil and 1 tablespoon butter to the skillet along with mushrooms and sauté over medium heat until just tender, 6 to 8 minutes. 4. Add the white wine, lemon juice, capers, and remaining ½ teaspoon salt to the skillet and bring to a boil, whisking to incorporate any little browned bits that have stuck to the bottom of the skillet. Reduce the heat to low and whisk in the final 2 tablespoons butter. 5. Return the browned chicken to skillet, cover, and simmer over low heat until the chicken is cooked through and the sauce has thickened, 5 to 6 more minutes. 6. Serve chicken and mushrooms warm over zucchini noodles, spooning the mushroom sauce over top and garnishing with chopped parsley.

Per Serving
Calories: 538 | Total Fat: 44g | Total Carbs: 8g | Net Carbs: 5g | Fiber: 3g | Protein: 30g | Sodium: 1128mg

Chicken Cutlets with Greek Salsa

Prep timePrep Time: 15 minutes | Cook Time: 15 minutes | Serves 2

- 2 tablespoons olive oil, divided
- Zest of ½ lemon
- 8 ounces (227 g) chicken cutlets, or chicken breast sliced through the middle to make 2 thin pieces
- ½ cup minced red onion (about ⅓ medium onion)
- 5 to 10 pitted Greek olives, minced (more or less depending on size and your taste)
- 1 tablespoon minced fresh oregano
- 1 ounce crumbled feta cheese
- ¼ teaspoon salt, plus additional to taste
- Juice of ½ lemon
- 1 cup cherry or grape tomatoes, halved or quartered (about 4 ounces / 113 g)
- 1 medium cucumber, peeled, seeded and diced (about 1 cup)
- 1 tablespoon minced fresh parsley
- 1 tablespoon minced fresh mint
- 1 tablespoon red wine vinegar

1. In a medium bowl, combine 1 tablespoon of olive oil, the salt, lemon zest, and lemon juice. Add the chicken and let it marinate while you make the salsa. 2. In a small bowl, combine the tomatoes, onion, cucumber, olives, parsley, oregano, mint, feta cheese, and red wine vinegar, and toss lightly. Cover and let rest in the refrigerator for at least 30 minutes. Taste the salsa before serving and add a pinch of salt or extra herbs if desired. 3. To cook the chicken, heat the remaining 1 tablespoon of olive oil in a large nonstick skillet over medium-high heat. Add the chicken pieces and cook for 3 to 6 minutes on each side, depending on the thickness. If the chicken sticks to the pan, it's not quite ready to flip. 4. When chicken is cooked through, top with the salsa and serve.

Per Serving
Calories: 357 | Total fat: 23g | Total carbs: 8g | Fiber: 2g | Sugar: 5g | Protein: 31g | Sodium: 202mg | Cholesterol: 90mg

Mediterranean Roasted Turkey Breast

Prep time: 15 minutes | Cook time: 6 to 8 hours | Serves 4

3 garlic cloves, minced
1 teaspoon dried oregano
½ teaspoon dried basil
½ teaspoon dried rosemary
¼ teaspoon dried dill
2 tablespoons extra-virgin olive oil
1 (4- to 6-pound) boneless or bone-in turkey breast
½ cup low-sodium chicken broth
1 cup sun-dried tomatoes (packaged, not packed in oil), chopped
1 teaspoon sea salt
½ teaspoon freshly ground black pepper
½ teaspoon dried parsley
½ teaspoon dried thyme
¼ teaspoon ground nutmeg
2 tablespoons freshly squeezed lemon juice
1 onion, chopped
4 ounces (113 g) whole Kalamata olives, pitted

1. In a small bowl, stir together the garlic, salt, oregano, pepper, basil, parsley, rosemary, thyme, dill, and nutmeg. 2. Drizzle the olive oil and lemon juice all over the turkey breast and generously season it with the garlic-spice mix. 3. In a slow cooker, combine the onion and chicken broth. Place the seasoned turkey breast on top of the onion. Top the turkey with the olives and sun-dried tomatoes. 4. Cover the cooker and cook for 6 to 8 hours on Low heat. 5. Slice or shred the turkey for serving.

Per Serving
Calories: 761 | Total fat: 55g | Sodium: 3,547mg | Carbohydrates: 20g | Fiber: 3g | Sugar: 10g | Protein: 83g

Moroccan-Spiced Chicken Thighs with Saffron Basmati Rice

Prep timePrep Time: 15 minutes | Cook Time: 15 minutes | Serves 2

For the chicken
½ teaspoon paprika
½ teaspoon cinnamon
¼ teaspoon garlic powder
¼ teaspoon coriander
10 ounces boneless, skinless chicken thighs (about 4 pieces)
For the rice
1 tablespoon olive oil
½ cup basmati rice
¼ teaspoon salt

½ teaspoon cumin
¼ teaspoon salt
¼ teaspoon ginger powder
⅛ teaspoon cayenne pepper (a pinch—or more if you like it spicy)

½ small onion, minced
2 pinches saffron
1 cup low-sodium chicken stock

To make the chicken:
1. Preheat the oven to 350°F (177°C) and set the rack to the middle position. 2. In a small bowl, combine the paprika, cumin, cinnamon, salt, garlic powder, ginger powder, coriander, and cayenne pepper. Add chicken thighs and toss, rubbing the spice mix into the chicken. 3. Place the chicken in a baking dish and roast it for 35 to 40 minutes, or until the chicken reaches an internal temperature of 160°F (74°C). Let the chicken rest for 5 minutes before serving.

To make the rice:
1. While the chicken is roasting, heat the oil in a sauté pan over medium-high heat. Add the onion and sauté for 5 minutes. 2. Add the rice, saffron, salt, and chicken stock. Cover the pot with a tight-fitting lid and reduce the heat to low. Let the rice simmer for 15 minutes, or until it is light and fluffy and the liquid has been absorbed.

Per Serving
Calories: 401 | Total fat: 10g | Total carbs: 41g | Fiber: 2g | Sugar: 1g | Protein: 37g | Sodium: 715mg | Cholesterol: 81mg

Chicken with Olives and Capers

Prep time: 10 minutes | Cook time: 6 to 8 hours | Serves 4

2 pounds (907g) bone-in, skin-on chicken thighs or legs
1 (3½ ounces) jar capers, with juice
1 garlic clove, minced
¼ teaspoon sea salt
2 tablespoons chopped fresh basil
1 (5¾ ounces) jar green olives, with juice
2 tablespoons red wine vinegar
1 teaspoon dried oregano
⅛ teaspoon freshly ground black pepper

1. Put the chicken in a slow cooker and top it with the olives and their juice and the capers and their juice. 2. Pour the vinegar over the chicken and sprinkle the garlic, oregano, salt, and pepper on top. 3. Cover the cooker and cook for 6 to 8 hours on Low heat. 4. Garnish with fresh basil for serving.

Per Serving
Calories: 553 | Total fat: 40g | Sodium: 1,073mg | Carbohydrates: 1g | Fiber: 1g | Sugar: 1g | Protein: 39g

Bomba Chicken with Chickpeas

Prep time: 10 minutes | Cook time: 30 minutes | Serves 4

2 pounds (907g) boneless, skinless chicken thighs
Freshly ground black pepper
1 onion, chopped
1 cup chicken broth
2 (15 ounces / 425-g) cans chickpeas, drained and rinsed
Sea salt
2 tablespoons olive oil, divided
3 garlic cloves, minced
1 tablespoon bomba sauce or harissa
¼ cup chopped fresh Italian parsley

1. Season the chicken thighs generously with salt and pepper. 2. In a large skillet, heat 1 tablespoon of olive oil over medium-high heat. Add the chicken and cook until browned, 2 to 3 minutes per side. Transfer the chicken to a plate and set aside. 3. In the same skillet, heat the remaining 1 tablespoon of olive oil. Add the onion and garlic and sauté for 4 to 5 minutes, until softened. Return the chicken to the skillet, then add the broth and bomba sauce. Bring to a boil, reduce the heat to low, cover, and simmer for 15 minutes, or until the chicken is cooked through. 4. Add the chickpeas and simmer for 5 minutes more. 5. Garnish with the parsley and serve.

Per Serving
Calories: 552 | Total fat: 19g | Total carbs: 37g | Sugar: 7g | Protein: 56g | Fiber: 10g | Sodium: 267mg

Chicken Avgolemono

Prep time: 10 minutes | Cook time: 50 minutes | Serves 4

1½ pounds (680 g) boneless, skinless chicken breasts
¾ cup dried Greek orzo
Juice of 2 lemons
Freshly ground black pepper
6 cups chicken broth, as needed
3 large eggs
Sea salt

1. Place the chicken in a stockpot and add enough broth to cover the chicken by 1 inch. Bring to a boil over high heat, then reduce the heat to low, cover, and simmer for 30 to 45 minutes, until the chicken is cooked through. Remove the chicken from the stockpot and set aside in a medium bowl. 2. Increase the heat to medium-high and bring the broth back to a boil. Add the orzo and cook for 7 to 10 minutes, until tender. 3. While the orzo is cooking, shred the chicken with two forks and return it to the pot when orzo is done. 4. Crack the eggs into a small bowl and whisk until frothy, then whisk in the lemon juice. While whisking continuously, slowly pour in 1 cup of the hot broth to temper the eggs. Pour the egg mixture back into the pot and stir. Simmer for 1 minute more, season with salt and pepper, and serve.

Per Serving
Calories: 391 | Total fat: 9g | Total carbs: 29g | Sugar: 1g | Protein: 46g | Fiber: 1g | Sodium: 171mg

Kale, Chickpea, and Chicken Stew

Prep time: 20 minutes | Cook time: 13 minutes | Serves 8

2 tablespoons light olive oil
1 medium yellow onion, peeled and chopped
2 cloves garlic, peeled and minced
2 sprigs thyme
2 (15 ounces / 425-g) cans chickpeas, drained and rinsed
2 cups low-sodium chicken broth
¼ cup chopped fresh parsley
2 large red bell peppers, seeded and chopped
4 cups chopped kale
3 medium tomatoes, seeded and chopped
1 pound (454 g) boneless, skinless chicken breast, cut into 1" pieces
½ cup tahini

1. Press the Sauté button on the Instant Pot® and heat oil. Add bell peppers and onion and sauté 5 minutes. Add kale and cook until just wilted, about 2 minutes. Add garlic and cook until fragrant, about 30 seconds. Add tomatoes and thyme. Press the Cancel button. 2. Add chicken, chickpeas, and broth. Stir well, then close lid, set steam release to Sealing, press the Manual button, and set time to 5 minutes. 3. When the timer beeps, let pressure release naturally for 15 minutes, then quick-release any remaining pressure until the float valve drops. Open lid and stir in tahini. Sprinkle with parsley and serve hot.

Per Serving
Calories: 310 | Fat: 14g | Protein: 25g | Sodium: 359mg | Fiber: 9g | Carbohydrates: 30g | Sugar: 6g

Chicken with Lemon Asparagus

Prep time: 10 minutes | Cook time: 13 minutes | Serves 4

2 tablespoons olive oil
½ teaspoon ground black pepper
¼ teaspoon smoked paprika
2 sprigs thyme
1 tablespoon grated lemon zest
¼ cup low-sodium chicken broth
¼ cup chopped fresh parsley
4 (6 ounces /170 g) boneless, skinless chicken breasts
¼ teaspoon salt
2 cloves garlic, peeled and minced
2 sprigs oregano
¼ cup lemon juice
1 bunch asparagus, trimmed
4 lemon wedges

1. Press Sauté on the Instant Pot® and heat oil. Season chicken with pepper, salt, and smoked paprika. Brown chicken on both sides, about 4 minutes per side. Add garlic, thyme, oregano, lemon zest, lemon juice, and chicken broth. Press the Cancel button. 2. Close lid, set steam release to Sealing, press the Manual button, and set time to 5 minutes. 3. When the timer beeps, quick-release the pressure until the float valve drops. Press the Cancel button and open lid. Transfer chicken breasts to a serving platter. Tent with foil to keep warm. 4. Add asparagus to the Instant Pot®. Close lid, set steam release to Sealing, press the Manual button, and set time to 0. When the timer beeps, quick-release the pressure until the float valve drops. Open lid and remove asparagus. Arrange asparagus around chicken and garnish with parsley and lemon wedges. Serve immediately.

Per Serving
Calories: 227 | Fat: 11g | Protein: 35g | Sodium: 426mg | Fiber: 0 | Carbohydrates: 0g | Sugar: 0g

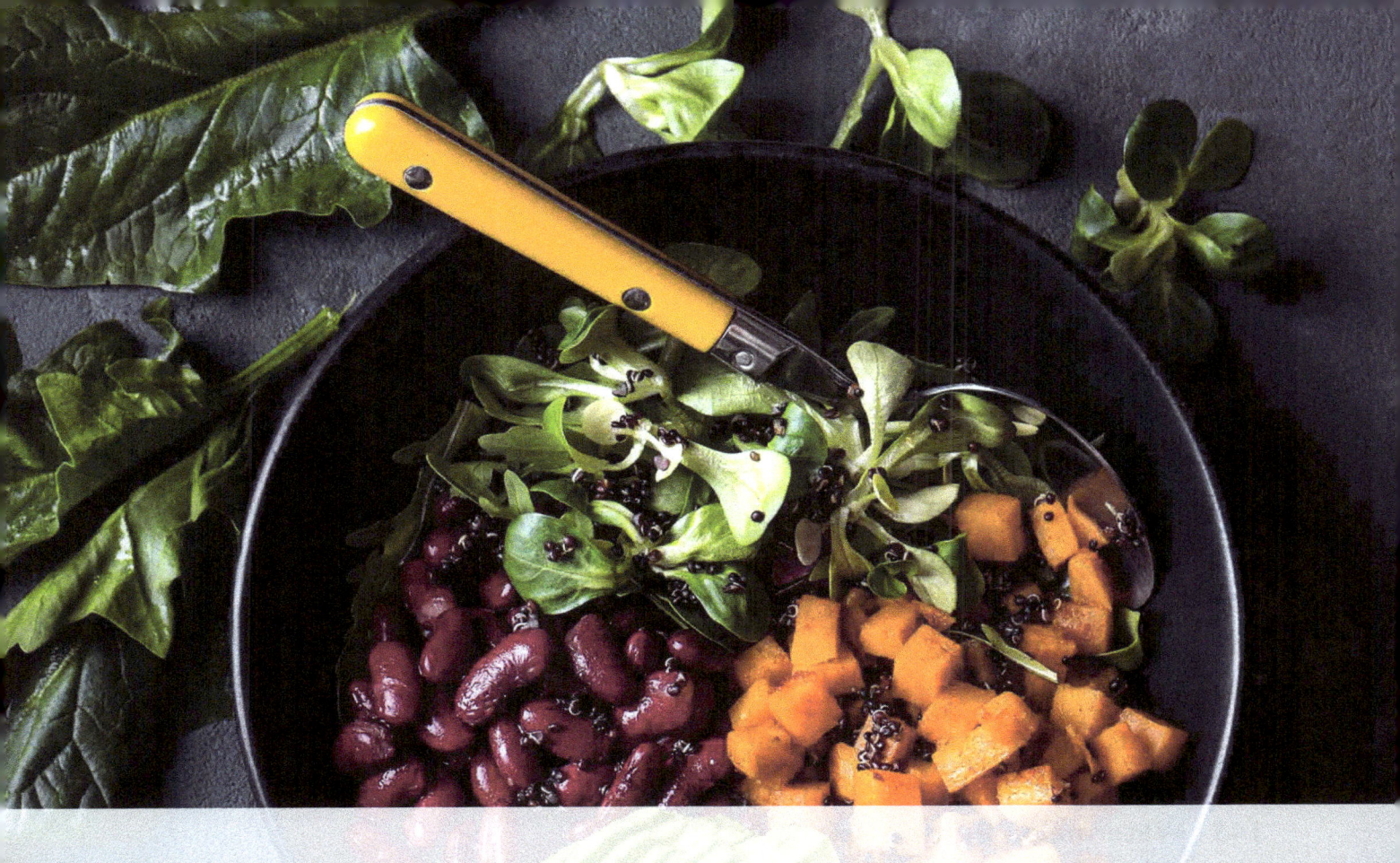

Chapter 10 Salads

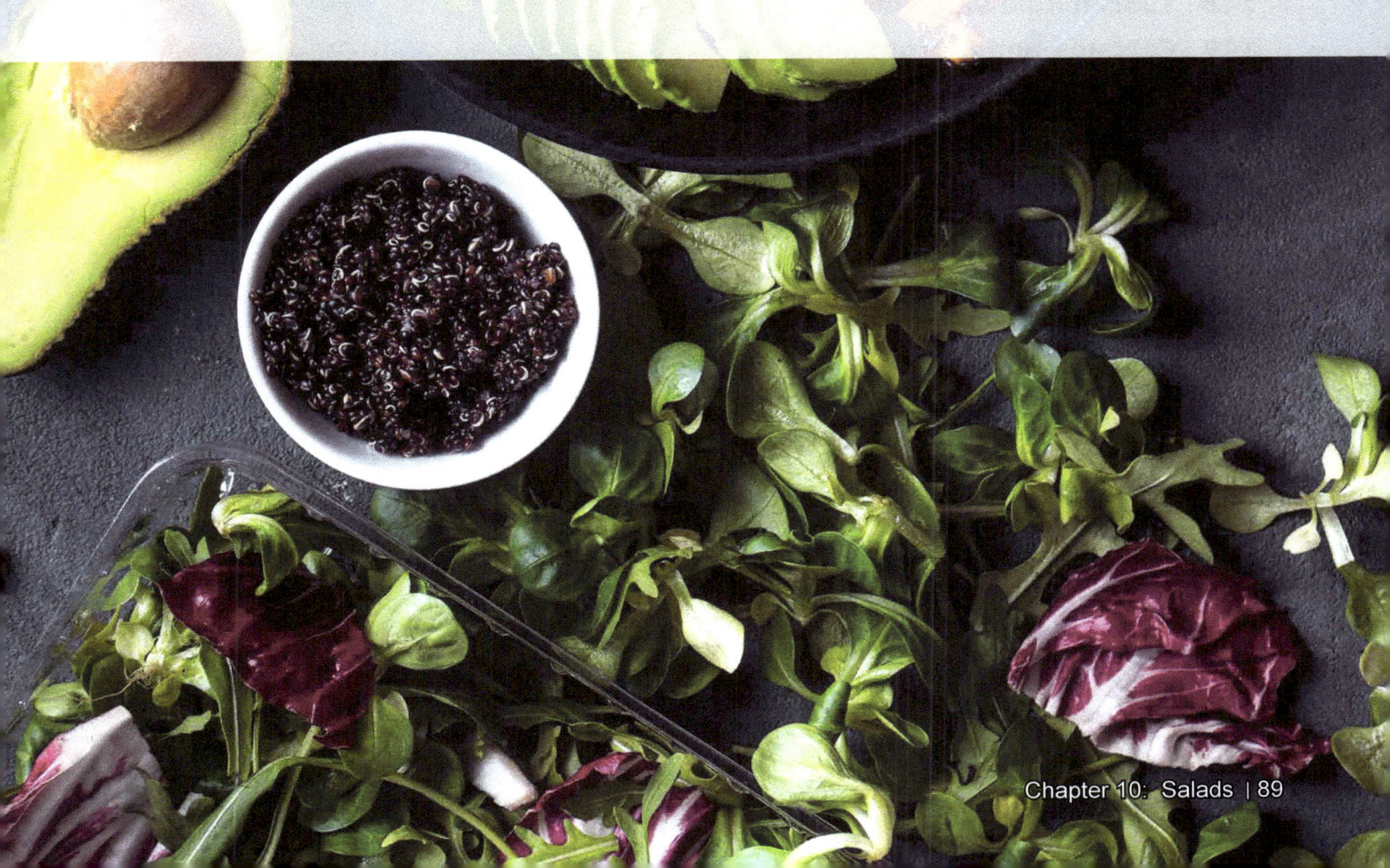

134 **Greek Village Salad**   91
135 **Greek Salad with Lemon-Oregano Vinaigrette**   91
136 **Cauliflower Tabbouleh Salad**   91
137 **Tabbouleh**   92
138 **Pistachio Quinoa Salad with Pomegranate Citrus Vinaigrette**   92
139 **Quinoa with Zucchini, Mint, and Pistachios**   93
140 **Superfood Salmon Salad Bowl**   93
141 **Turkish Shepherd'S Salad**   94
142 **Classic Tabouli**   94
143 **No-Mayo Florence Tuna Salad**   94
144 **Taverna-Style Greek Salad**   95
145 **Watermelon Burrata Salad**   95
146 **Mediterranean Quinoa and Garbanzo Salad**   95
147 **Roasted Golden Beet, Avocado, and Watercress Salad**   96
148 **Tuscan Kale Salad with Anchovies**   96
149 **Cabbage and Carrot Salad**   96
150 **Roasted Cauliflower and Arugula Salad with Pomegranate and Pine Nuts**   97
151 **Wild Rice Salad with Chickpeas and Pickled Radish**   97
152 **Toasted Pita Bread Salad**   98
153 **Traditional Greek Salad**   98
154 **Marinated Greek Salad with Oregano and Goat Cheese**   99
155 **Mediterranean Pasta Salad**   99

Greek Village Salad

Prep time: 10 minutes | Cook time: 0 minutes | Serves 4

5 large tomatoes, cut into medium chunks
1 English cucumber, peeled and cut into medium chunks
1 cup kalamata olives, for topping
¼ lemon
2 red onions, cut into medium chunks or sliced
2 green bell peppers, cut into medium chunks
¼ cup extra-virgin olive oil, plus extra for drizzling
¼ teaspoon dried oregano, plus extra for garnish
4 ounces (113 g) Greek feta cheese, sliced

1. In a large bowl, mix the tomatoes, onions, cucumber, bell peppers, olive oil, olives, and oregano. 2. Divide the vegetable mixture evenly among four bowls and top each with a squirt of lemon juice and 1 slice of feta. Drizzle with olive oil, garnish with oregano, and serve.

Per Serving
Calories: 315 | Total fat: 24g | Total carbs: 21g | Sugar: 12g | Protein: 8g | Fiber: 6g | Sodium: 524mg

Greek Salad with Lemon-Oregano Vinaigrette

Prep time: 15 minutes | Cook time: 15 minutes | Serves 8

½ red onion, thinly sliced
3 tablespoons fresh lemon juice or red wine vinegar
1 teaspoon chopped fresh oregano or ½ teaspoon dried
¼ teaspoon kosher salt
1 large English cucumber, peeled, seeded (if desired), and diced
¼ cup chopped fresh flat-leaf parsley
¼ cup extra-virgin olive oil
1 clove garlic, minced
½ teaspoon ground black pepper
4 tomatoes, cut into large chunks
1 large yellow or red bell pepper, chopped
½ cup pitted kalamata or Niçoise olives, halved
4 ounces (113 g) Halloumi or feta cheese, cut into ½" cubes

1. In a medium bowl, soak the onion in enough water to cover for 10 minutes. 2. In a small bowl, combine the oil, lemon juice or vinegar, garlic, oregano, black pepper, and salt. 3. Drain the onion and add to a large bowl with the tomatoes, cucumber, bell pepper, olives, and parsley. Gently toss to mix the vegetables. 4. Pour the vinaigrette over the salad. Add the cheese and toss again to distribute. 5. Serve immediately, or chill for up to 30 minutes.

Per Serving
calories:190 | protein: 5g | carbohydrates: 8g | sugars: 3g | total fat: 16g | saturated fat: 4g | fiber: 2g | sodium: 554mg

Cauliflower Tabbouleh Salad

Prep time: 15 minutes | Cook time: 0 minutes | Serves 4

¼ cup extra-virgin olive oil
Zest of 1 lemon
½ teaspoon ground turmeric
¼ teaspoon ground cumin
⅛ teaspoon ground cinnamon
1 English cucumber, diced
1 cup fresh parsley, chopped
¼ cup lemon juice
¾ teaspoon kosher salt
¼ teaspoon ground coriander
¼ teaspoon black pepper
1 pound (454 g) riced cauliflower
12 cherry tomatoes, halved
½ cup fresh mint, chopped

1. In a large bowl, whisk together the olive oil, lemon juice, lemon zest, salt, turmeric, coriander, cumin, black pepper, and cinnamon. 2. Add the riced cauliflower to the bowl and mix well. Add in the cucumber, tomatoes, parsley, and mint and gently mix together.

Per Serving
Calories: 180 | Fat: 15g | Protein: 4g | Carbs: 12g | Sugars: 5g | Fiber: 5g | Sodium:260 mg | Cholesterol: 0mg

Tabbouleh

Prep time: 15 minutes | Cook time: 12 minutes | Serves 4 to 6

1 cup water
½ English cucumber, quartered lengthwise and sliced
2 scallions, chopped
2 cups coarsely chopped fresh Italian parsley
1 garlic clove
Sea salt
½ cup dried bulgur
2 tomatoes on the vine, diced
Juice of 1 lemon
⅓ cup coarsely chopped fresh mint leaves
¼ cup extra-virgin olive oil
Freshly ground black pepper

1. In a medium saucepan, combine the water and bulgur and bring to a boil over medium heat. Reduce the heat to low, cover, and cook until the bulgur is tender, about 12 minutes. Drain off any excess liquid, fluff the bulgur with a fork, and set aside to cool. 2. In a large bowl, toss together the bulgur, cucumber, tomatoes, scallions, and lemon juice. 3. In a food processor, combine the parsley, mint, and garlic and process until finely chopped. 4. Add the chopped herb mixture to the bulgur mixture and stir to combine. Add the olive oil and stir to incorporate. 5. Season with salt and pepper and serve.

Per Serving
Calories: 215 | Total fat: 14g | Total carbs: 21g | Sugar: 3g | Protein: 4g | Fiber: 5g | Sodium: 66mg

Pistachio Quinoa Salad with Pomegranate Citrus Vinaigrette

Prep time: 15 minutes | Cook time: 15 minutes | Serves 6

For the Quinoa:
1½ cups water
¼ teaspoon kosher salt
1 cup quinoa

For the Dressing:
1 cup extra-virgin olive oil
½ cup freshly squeezed orange juice
1 teaspoon pure maple syrup
½ teaspoon ground sumac
¼ teaspoon freshly ground black pepper
½ cup pomegranate juice
1 small shallot, minced
1 teaspoon za'atar
½ teaspoon kosher salt

For the Salad:
3 cups baby spinach
½ cup fresh mint, coarsely chopped
¼ cup pistachios, shelled and toasted
¼ cup crumbled blue cheese
½ cup fresh parsley, coarsely chopped
Approximately ¾ cup pomegranate seeds, or 2 pomegranates

To Make the Quinoa:
Bring the water, quinoa, and salt to a boil in a small saucepan. Reduce the heat and cover; simmer for 10 to 12 minutes. Fluff with a fork.

To Make the Dressing:
1. In a medium bowl, whisk together the olive oil, pomegranate juice, orange juice, shallot, maple syrup, za'atar, sumac, salt, and black pepper. 2. In a large bowl, add about ½ cup of dressing. 3. Store the remaining dressing in a glass jar or airtight container and refrigerate. The dressing can be kept up to 2 weeks. Let the chilled dressing reach room temperature before using.

To Make the Salad:
1. Combine the spinach, parsley, and mint in the bowl with the dressing and toss gently together. 5 Add the quinoa. Toss gently. 2. Add the pomegranate seeds. 3. Or, if using whole pomegranates: Cut the pomegranates in half. Fill a large bowl with water and hold the pomegranate half, cut side-down. Using a wooden spoon, hit the back of the pomegranate so the seeds fall into the water. Immerse the pomegranate in the water and gently pull out any remaining seeds. Repeat with the remaining pomegranate. Skim the white pith off the top of the water. Drain the seeds and add them to the greens. 8 Add the pistachios and cheese and toss gently.

Per Serving
Calories: 300 | Fat: 19g | Protein: 8g | Carbs: 28g | Sugars: 8g | Fiber: 5g | Sodium: 225mg | Cholesterol: 6mg

Quinoa with Zucchini, Mint, and Pistachios

Prep time: 20 to 30 minutes | Cook time: 20 minutes | Serves 4

For the Quinoa:
1½ cups water
¼ teaspoon kosher salt

1 cup quinoa

For the Salad:
2 tablespoons extra-virgin olive oil
6 small radishes, sliced
¾ teaspoon kosher salt
2 garlic cloves, sliced
2 tablespoons lemon juice
¼ cup fresh basil, chopped

1 zucchini, thinly sliced into rounds
1 shallot, julienned
¼ teaspoon freshly ground black pepper
Zest of 1 lemon
¼ cup fresh mint, chopped
¼ cup pistachios, shelled and toasted

To Make the Quinoa:
Bring the water, quinoa, and salt to a boil in a medium saucepan. Reduce to a simmer, cover, and cook for 10 to 12 minutes. Fluff with a fork.

To Make the Salad:
1. Heat the olive oil in a large skillet or sauté pan over medium-high heat. Add the zucchini, radishes, shallot, salt, and black pepper, and sauté for 7 to 8 minutes. Add the garlic and cook 30 seconds to 1 minute more. 2. In a large bowl, combine the lemon zest and lemon juice. Add the quinoa and mix well. Add the cooked zucchini mixture and mix well. Add the mint, basil, and pistachios and gently mix.

Per Serving
Calories: 220 | Fat: 12g | Protein: 6g | Carbs: 25g | Sugars: 5g | Fiber: 5g | Sodium: 295mg | Cholesterol: 0mg

Superfood Salmon Salad Bowl

Prep time: 5 minutes | Cook time: 10 minutes | Serves 2

Salmon
2 fillets (250 g/8.8 ounces) wild salmon
2 teaspoons (10 ml) extra-virgin avocado oil

Salt and black pepper, to taste

Dressing
1 tablespoon (9 g/0.3 ounces) capers
1 tablespoon (15 ml) apple cider vinegar
or fresh lemon juice
Salt and black pepper, to taste

1 teaspoon Dijon or whole-grain mustard
3 tablespoons (45 ml) extra-virgin olive oil
1 teaspoon coconut aminos

Salad
½ medium (200 g/7 ounces) cucumber, diced
½ small (40 g/1.4 ounces) red bell pepper, sliced
⅓ cup (33 g/1.2 ounces) pitted Kalamata olives, halved
1 medium (150 g/5.3 ounces) avocado, diced
1 tablespoon (8 g/0.3 ounces) pumpkin seeds
1 tablespoon (9 g/0.3 ounces) sunflower seeds

1 cup (50 g/1.8 ounces) sugar snap peas, sliced into matchsticks
2 sun-dried tomatoes (14 g/0.5 ounces), chopped
3 tablespoons (12 g/0.4 ounces) chopped fresh herbs, such as dill, chives, parsley, and/or basil

1. To make the salmon: Season the salmon with salt and pepper. Heat a pan greased with the avocado oil over medium heat. Add the salmon, skin-side down, and cook for 4 to 5 minutes. Flip and cook for 1 to 2 minutes or until cooked through. Remove from the heat and transfer to a plate to cool. Remove the skin from the salmon and flake into chunks. 2. To make the dressing: Mix all the dressing ingredients together in a small bowl. Set aside. 3. To make the salad: Place the cucumber, sugar snap peas, bell pepper, olives, sun-dried tomatoes, avocado, and herbs in a mixing bowl, and combine well. Add the flaked salmon. Dry-fry the seeds in a pan placed over medium-low heat until lightly golden. Allow to cool, then add to the bowl. Drizzle with the prepared dressing and serve. This salad can be stored in the fridge for up to 1 day.

Per Serving
Total carbs: 17.6 g | Fiber: 8.6 g | Net Carbs: 9 g | Protein: 31 g | Fat: 53.6 g (of which saturated: 7.8 g) | Calories: 660

Turkish Shepherd'S Salad

Prep time: 15 minutes | Cook time: 0 minutes | Serves 6

¼ cup extra-virgin olive oil
2 tablespoons lemon juice
¼ teaspoon ground black pepper
2 cucumbers, seeded and chopped
1 green bell pepper, seeded and chopped
⅓ cup pitted black olives (such as kalamata), halved
¼ cup chopped fresh mint
6 ounces (170 g) feta cheese, cubed
2 tablespoons apple cider vinegar
½ teaspoon kosher salt
3 plum tomatoes, seeded and chopped
1 red bell pepper, seeded and chopped
1 small red onion, chopped
½ cup chopped fresh flat-leaf parsley
¼ cup chopped fresh dill

1. In a small bowl, whisk together the oil, vinegar, lemon juice, salt, and black pepper. 2. In a large serving bowl, combine the tomatoes, cucumber, bell peppers, onion, olives, parsley, mint, and dill. Pour the dressing over the salad, toss gently, and sprinkle with the cheese.

Per Serving
calories:238 | protein: 6g | carbohydrates: 10g | sugars: 5g | total fat: 20g | saturated fat: 6g | fiber:2g | sodium: 806mg

Classic Tabouli

Prep time: 30 minutes | Cook time: 0 minutes | Serves 8 to 10

1 cup bulgur wheat, grind #1
2 cups ripe tomato, finely diced
½ cup lemon juice
1½ teaspoons salt
4 cups Italian parsley, finely chopped
1 cup green onion, finely chopped
½ cup extra-virgin olive oil
1 teaspoon dried mint

1. Before you chop the vegetables, put the bulgur in a small bowl. Rinse with water, drain, and let stand in the bowl while you prepare the other ingredients. 2. Put the parsley, tomatoes, green onion, and bulgur into a large bowl. 3. In a small bowl, whisk together the lemon juice, olive oil, salt, and mint. 4. Pour the dressing over the tomato, onion, and bulgur mixture, tossing everything together. Add additional salt to taste. Serve immediately or store in the fridge for up to 2 days.

Per Serving
Calories: 207 | Protein: 4g | Total Carbohydrates: 20g | Sugars: 1g | Fiber: 5g | Total Fat: 14g | Saturated Fat: 2g | Cholesterol: 0mg | Sodium: 462mg

No-Mayo Florence Tuna Salad

Prep time: 10 minutes | Cook time: 0 minutes | Serves 4

4 cups spring mix greens
2 (5 ounces) cans water-packed, white albacore tuna, drained (I prefer Wild Planet brand)
¼ cup sliced pitted kalamata olives
3 tablespoons extra-virgin olive oil
2 or 3 leaves thinly chopped fresh sweet basil
Kosher salt
1 (15 ounces / 425-g) can cannellini beans, drained
⅔ cup crumbled feta cheese
½ cup thinly sliced sun-dried tomatoes
¼ cup thinly sliced scallions, both green and white parts
½ teaspoon dried cilantro
1 lime, zested and juiced
Freshly ground black pepper

1. In a large bowl, combine greens, beans, tuna, feta, tomatoes, olives, scallions, olive oil, cilantro, basil, and lime juice and zest. Season with salt and pepper, mix, and enjoy!

Per Serving
Calories: 355 | Protein: 22g | Total Carbohydrates: 25g | Sugars: 5g | Fiber: 8g | Total Fat: 19g | Saturated Fat: 5g | Cholesterol: 47mg | Sodium: 744mg

Taverna-Style Greek Salad

Prep time: 20 minutes | Cook time: 0 minutes | Serves 4

4 to 5 (400 g/14.1 ounces) medium tomatoes, roughly chopped
1 medium (120 g/4.2 ounces) green bell pepper, sliced
16 pitted (48 g/1.7 ounces) Kalamata olives
1 teaspoon dried oregano or fresh herbs of your choice, such as parsley, cilantro, chives, or basil, divided
Optional: salt, pepper, and fresh oregano, for garnish
1 large (300 g/10.6 ounces) cucumber, peeled and roughly chopped
1 small (60 g/2.1 ounces) red onion, sliced
¼ cup (35 g/1.2 ounces) capers, or more olives
½ cup (120 ml) extra-virgin olive oil, divided
1 pack (200 g/7 ounces) feta cheese

1. Place the vegetables in a large serving bowl. Add the olives, capers, feta, half of the dried oregano and half of the olive oil. Mix to combine. Place the whole piece of feta cheese on top, sprinkle with the remaining dried oregano, and drizzle with the remaining olive oil. Season to taste and serve immediately, or store in the fridge for up to 1 day.

Per Serving
Total carbs: 11.3 g | Fiber: 3.3 g | Net Carbs: 8 g | Protein: 9.3 g | Fat: 41.3 g (of which saturated: 12.6) | Calories: 443

Watermelon Burrata Salad

Prep time: 10 minutes | Cook time: 0 minutes | Serves 4

2 cups cubes or chunks watermelon
1 small red onion or 2 shallots, thinly sliced into half-moons
¼ cup balsamic vinegar
1 tablespoon lemon zest
Salt and freshly ground black pepper, to taste
1½ cups small burrata cheese balls, cut into medium chunks
¼ cup olive oil
4 fresh basil leaves, sliced chiffonade-style (roll up leaves of basil, and slice into thin strips)

1. In a large bowl, mix all the ingredients. Refrigerate until chilled before serving.

Per Serving (1 cup)
Calories: 224 | Fat: 14g | Protein: 14g | Carbs: 12g | Sugars: 8g | Fiber: 1g | Sodium: 560mg | Cholesterol: 8mg

Mediterranean Quinoa and Garbanzo Salad

Prep time: 10 minutes | Cook time: 30 minutes | Serves 8

4 cups water
2 teaspoons salt, divided
1 (16 ounces / 454 g) can garbanzo beans, rinsed and drained
1 teaspoon freshly ground black pepper
2 cups red or yellow quinoa
1 cup thinly sliced onions (red or white)
⅓ cup extra-virgin olive oil
¼ cup lemon juice

1. In a 3-quart pot over medium heat, bring the water to a boil. 2. Add the quinoa and 1 teaspoon of salt to the pot. Stir, cover, and let cook over low heat for 15 to 20 minutes. 3. Turn off the heat, fluff the quinoa with a fork, cover again, and let stand for 5 to 10 more minutes. 4. Put the cooked quinoa, onions, and garbanzo beans in a large bowl. 5. In a separate small bowl, whisk together the olive oil, lemon juice, remaining 1 teaspoon of salt, and black pepper. 6. Add the dressing to the quinoa mixture and gently toss everything together. Serve warm or cold.

Per Serving
Calories: 318 | Protein: 9g | Total Carbohydrates: 43g | Sugars: 6g | Fiber: 6g | Total Fat: 13g | Saturated Fat: 1g | Cholesterol: 0mg | Sodium: 585mg

Roasted Golden Beet, Avocado, and Watercress Salad

Prep time: 15 minutes | Cook time: 1 hour | Serves 4

1 bunch (about 1½ pounds / 680 g) golden beets
1 tablespoon white wine vinegar
¼ teaspoon freshly ground black pepper
1 avocado, peeled, pitted, and diced
¼ cup walnuts, toasted
1 tablespoon extra-virgin olive oil
½ teaspoon kosher salt
1 bunch (about 4 ounces / 113 g) watercress
¼ cup crumbled feta cheese
1 tablespoon fresh chives, chopped

1. Preheat the oven to 425°F (218°C). Wash and trim the beets (cut an inch above the beet root, leaving the long tail if desired), then wrap each beet individually in foil. Place the beets on a baking sheet and roast until fully cooked, 45 to 60 minutes depending on the size of each beet. Start checking at 45 minutes; if easily pierced with a fork, the beets are cooked. 2. Remove the beets from the oven and allow them to cool. Under cold running water, slough off the skin. Cut the beets into bite-size cubes or wedges. 3. In a large bowl, whisk together the olive oil, vinegar, salt, and black pepper. Add the watercress and beets and toss well. Add the avocado, feta, walnuts, and chives and mix gently.

Per Serving
Calories: 235 | Fat: 16g | Protein: 6g | Carbs: 21g | Sugars: 12g | Fiber: 8g | Sodium: 365mg | Cholesterol: 8mg

Tuscan Kale Salad with Anchovies

Prep time: 15 minutes | Cook time: 0 minutes | Serves 4

1 large bunch lacinato or dinosaur kale
1 cup shaved or coarsely shredded fresh Parmesan cheese
2 to 3 tablespoons freshly squeezed lemon juice (from 1 large lemon)
¼ cup toasted pine nuts
¼ cup extra-virgin olive oil
8 anchovy fillets, roughly chopped
2 teaspoons red pepper flakes (optional)

1. Remove the rough center stems from the kale leaves and roughly tear each leaf into about 4-by-1-inch strips. Place the torn kale in a large bowl and add the pine nuts and cheese. 2. In a small bowl, whisk together the olive oil, anchovies, lemon juice, and red pepper flakes (if using). Drizzle over the salad and toss to coat well. Let sit at room temperature 30 minutes before serving, tossing again just prior to serving.

Per Serving
Calories: 337 | Total Fat: 25g | Total Carbs: 12g | Net Carbs: 10g | Fiber: 2g | Protein: 16g | Sodium: 603mg

Cabbage and Carrot Salad

Prep time: 10 minutes | Cook time: 0 minutes | Serves 3

½ medium head cabbage, thinly sliced, rinsed, and drained
3 tablespoons fresh lemon juice
¼ teaspoons freshly ground black pepper
8 Kalamata olives, pitted
3 medium carrots, peeled and shredded
4 tablespoons extra virgin olive oil
½ teaspoons salt
1 garlic clove, minced

1. Place the cabbage and carrots in a large bowl and toss. 2. In a jar or small bowl, combine the olive oil, lemon juice, salt, black pepper, and garlic. Whisk or shake to combine. 3. Pour the dressing over the salad and toss. (Note that it will reduce in volume.) 4. Scatter the olives over the salad just before serving. Store covered in the refrigerator for up to 2 days.

Per Serving
Calories: 268 | Total fat: 21g | Saturated fat: 3g | Carbohydrate: 16g | Protein: 3g

Roasted Cauliflower and Arugula Salad with Pomegranate and Pine Nuts

Prep time: 20 minutes | Cook time: 20 minutes | Serves 4

1 head cauliflower, trimmed and cut into 1-inch florets
1 teaspoon ground cumin
¼ teaspoon freshly ground black pepper
⅓ cup pomegranate seeds
2 tablespoons extra-virgin olive oil, plus more for drizzling (optional)
½ teaspoon kosher salt
5 ounces (142 g) arugula
¼ cup pine nuts, toasted

1. Preheat the oven to 425°F (218°C). Line a baking sheet with parchment paper or foil. 2. In a large bowl, combine the cauliflower, olive oil, cumin, salt, and black pepper. Spread in a single layer on the prepared baking sheet and roast for 20 minutes, tossing halfway through. 3. Divide the arugula among 4 plates. Top with the cauliflower, pomegranate seeds, and pine nuts. 4. Serve with a simple drizzle of olive oil.

Per Serving
Calories: 190 | Fat: 14g | Protein: 6g | Carbs: 16g | Sugars: 7g | Fiber: 6g | Sodium: 210mg | Cholesterol: 0mg

Wild Rice Salad with Chickpeas and Pickled Radish

Prep time: 20 minutes | Cook time: 45 minutes | Serves 6

For the Rice:
1 cup water
¼ teaspoon kosher salt
4 ounces (113 g) wild rice

For the Pickled Radish:
1 bunch radishes (6 to 8 small), thinly sliced
½ teaspoon kosher salt
½ cup white wine vinegar

For the Dressing:
2 tablespoons extra-virgin olive oil
½ teaspoon pure maple syrup
¼ teaspoon freshly ground black pepper
2 tablespoons white wine vinegar
½ teaspoon kosher salt

For the Salad:
1 (15 ounces / 425-g) can no-salt-added or low-sodium chickpeas, rinsed and drained
¼ cup crumbled feta cheese
2 tablespoons fresh dill, chopped
1 bulb fennel, diced
¼ cup walnuts, chopped and toasted
¼ cup currants

To Make the Rice:
Bring the water, rice, and salt to a boil in a medium saucepan. Cover, reduce the heat, and simmer for 45 minutes.
To Make the Pickled Radish:
In a medium bowl, combine the radishes, vinegar, and salt. Let sit for 15 to 30 minutes.
To Make the Dressing:
1. In a large bowl, whisk together the olive oil, vinegar, maple syrup, salt, and black pepper. To Make the Salad: 1 While still warm, add the rice to the bowl with the dressing and mix well. 2. Add the chickpeas, fennel, walnuts, feta, currants, and dill. Mix well. 3. Garnish with the pickled radishes before serving.

Per Serving
Calories: 310 | Fat: 16g | Protein: 10g | Carbs: 36g | Sugars: 11g | Fiber: 7g | Sodium: 400mg | Cholesterol: 8mg

Toasted Pita Bread Salad

Prep time: 10 minutes | Cook time: 0 minutes | Serves 4

For the dressing
½ cup lemon juice
1 small clove garlic, minced
½ teaspoon ground sumac

½ cup olive oil
1 teaspoon salt
¼ teaspoon freshly ground black pepper

For the salad
2 cups shredded romaine lettuce
2 medium tomatoes, diced
¼ cup chopped fresh mint leaves
1 bunch scallions, thinly sliced
Ground sumac for garnish

1 large or 2 small cucumbers, seeded and diced
½ cup chopped fresh flat-leaf parsley leaves
1 small green bell pepper, diced
2 whole-wheat pita bread rounds, toasted and broken into quarter-sized pieces

1. To make the dressing, whisk together the lemon juice, olive oil, garlic, salt, sumac, and pepper in a small bowl. 2. To make the salad, in a large bowl, combine the lettuce, cucumber, tomatoes, parsley, mint, bell pepper, scallions, and pita bread. Toss to combine. Add the dressing and toss again to coat well. 3. Serve immediately sprinkled with sumac.

Per Serving
Calories: 359 | Total Fat: 27g | Saturated Fat: 4g | Carbs: 29g | Protein: 6g | Sodium: 777mg | Fiber: 6g

Traditional Greek Salad

Prep time: 10 minutes | Cook time: 0 minutes | Serves 4

2 large English cucumbers
1 green bell pepper, cut into 1- to 1½-inch chunks
4 ounces (113 g) pitted Kalamata olives
2 tablespoons freshly squeezed lemon juice
1 tablespoon chopped fresh oregano or
1 teaspoon dried oregano

4 Roma tomatoes, quartered
¼ small red onion, thinly sliced
¼ cup extra-virgin olive oil
1 tablespoon red wine vinegar
¼ teaspoon freshly ground black pepper
4 ounces (113 g) crumbled traditional feta cheese

1. Cut the cucumbers in half lengthwise and then into ½-inch-thick half-moons. Place in a large bowl. 2. Add the quartered tomatoes, bell pepper, red onion, and olives. 3. In a small bowl, whisk together the olive oil, lemon juice, vinegar, oregano, and pepper. Drizzle over the vegetables and toss to coat. 4. Divide between salad plates and top each with 1 ounce of feta.

Per Serving
Calories: 278 | Total Fat: 22g | Total Carbs: 12g | Net Carbs: 8g | Fiber: 4g | Protein: 8g | Sodium: 572mg

Marinated Greek Salad with Oregano and Goat Cheese

Prep time: 10 minutes | Cook time: 0 minutes | Serves 4

½ cup white wine vinegar
1 teaspoon crumbled dried Greek oregano
¼ teaspoon freshly ground black pepper
4 to 6 long, skinny red or yellow banana peppers or other mild peppers
2 ounces crumbled goat cheese or feta

1 small garlic clove, minced
½ teaspoon salt
2 Persian cucumbers, sliced thinly
1 medium red onion, cut into rings
1 pint mixed small heirloom tomatoes, halved

1. In a large, nonreactive (glass, ceramic, or plastic) bowl, whisk together the vinegar, garlic, oregano, salt, and pepper. Add the cucumbers, peppers, and onion and toss to mix. Cover and refrigerate for at least 1 hour. 2. Add the tomatoes to the bowl and toss to coat. Serve topped with the cheese.

Per Serving
Calories: 98 | Total Fat: 4g | Saturated Fat: 2g | Carbs: 13g | Protein: 4g | Sodium: 460mg | Fiber: 3g

Mediterranean Pasta Salad

Prep time: 20 minutes | Cook time: 15 minutes | Serves 4

4 cups dried farfalle (bow-tie) pasta
⅔ cup water-packed artichoke hearts, drained and diced
½ red bell pepper, diced
½ English cucumber, quartered lengthwise and cut into ½-inch pieces
Sea salt
½ cup crumbled feta cheese

1 cup canned chickpeas, drained and rinsed
½ red onion, thinly sliced
1 cup packed baby spinach
1 Roma (plum) tomato, diced
⅓ cup extra-virgin olive oil
Juice of ½ lemon
Freshly ground black pepper

1. Fill a large saucepan three-quarters full with water and bring to a boil over high heat. Add the pasta and cook according to the package directions until al dente, about 15 minutes. Drain the pasta and run it under cold water to stop the cooking process and cool. 2. While the pasta is cooking, in a large bowl, mix the chickpeas, artichoke hearts, onion, spinach, bell pepper, tomato, and cucumber. 3. Add the pasta to the bowl with the vegetables. Add the olive oil and lemon juice and season with salt and black pepper. Mix well. 4. Top the salad with the feta and serve.

Per Serving
Calories: 702 | Total fat: 25g | Total carbs: 99g | Sugar: 8g | Protein: 22g | Fiber: 10g | Sodium: 207mg

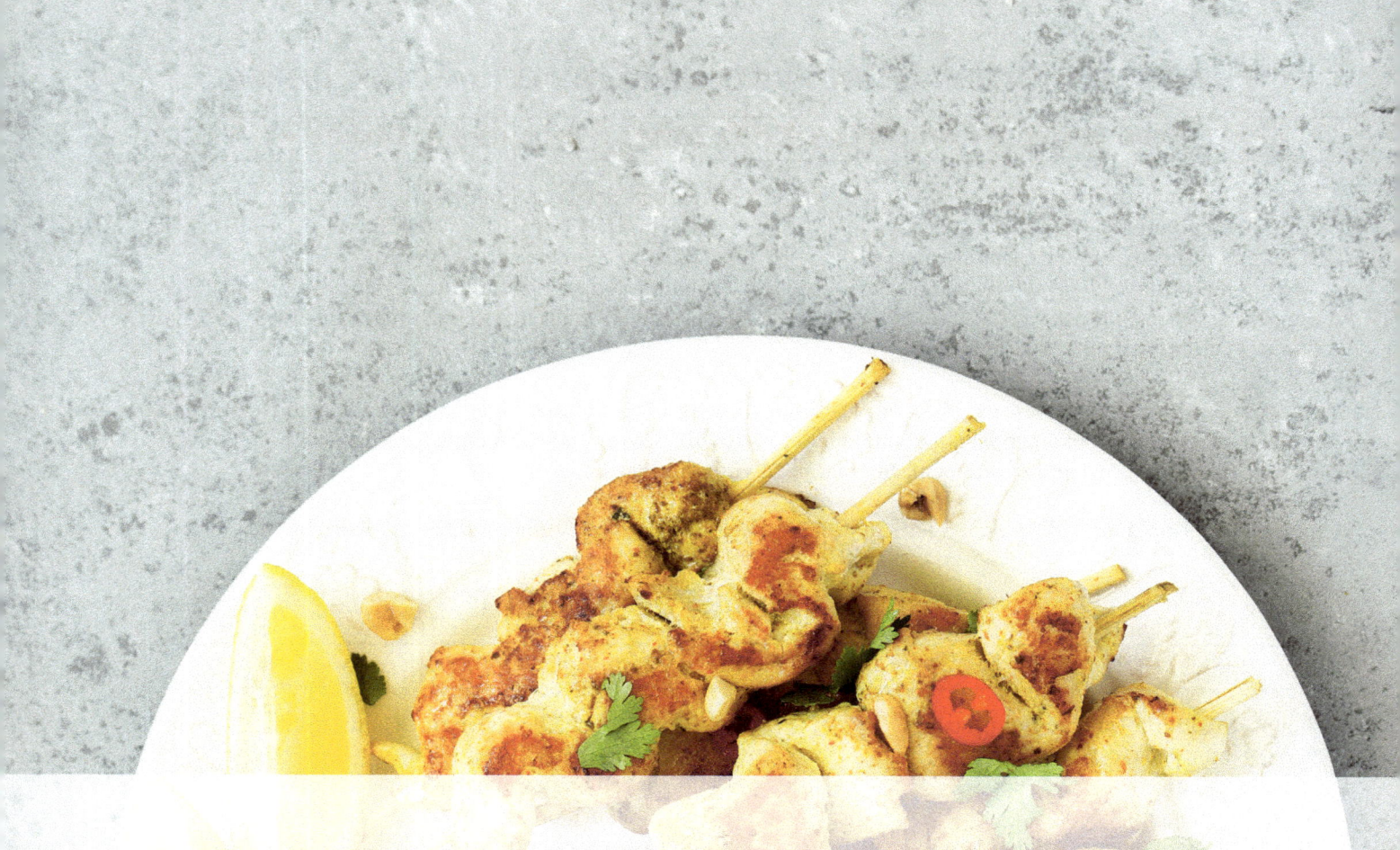

Chapter 11   Snacks and Appetizers

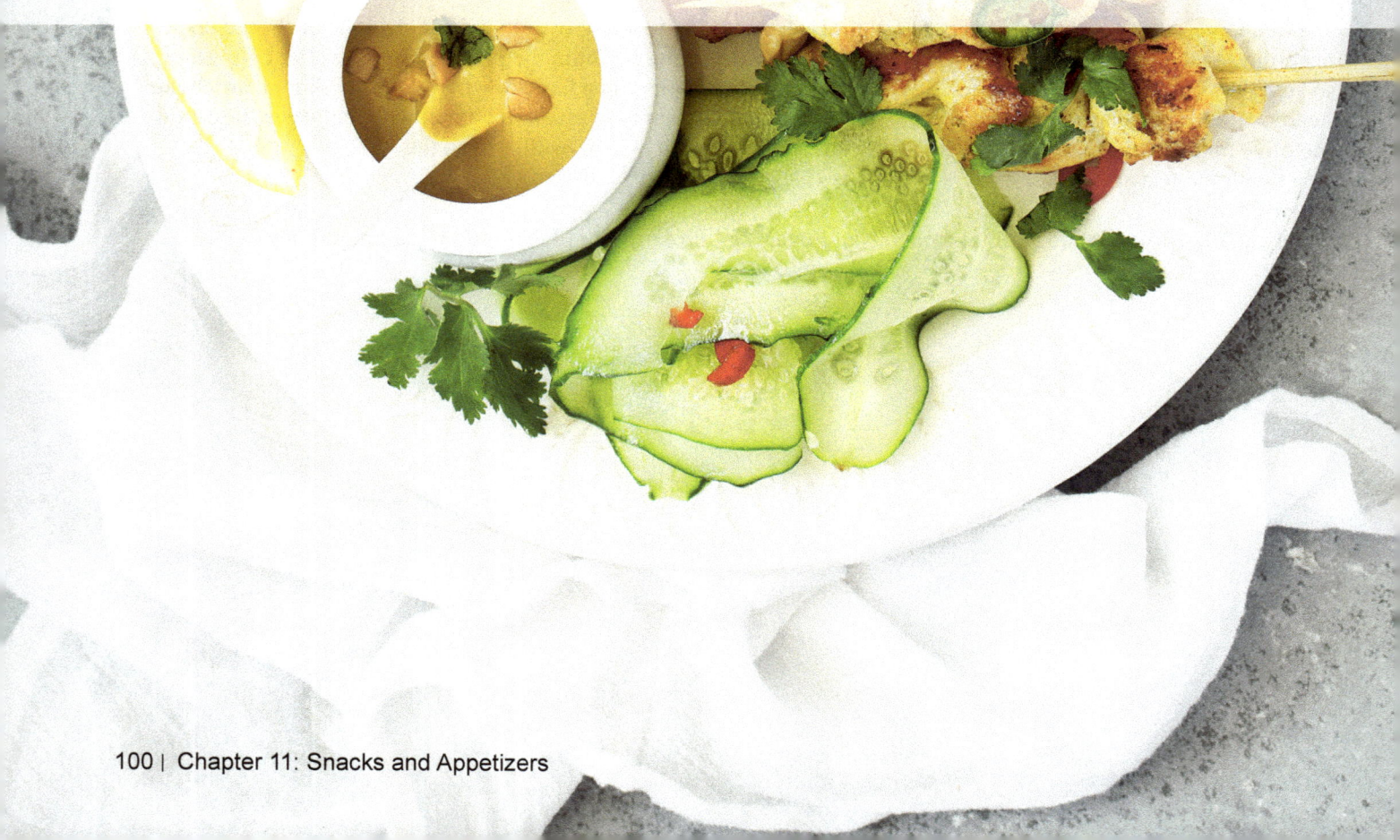

156 **Goat'S Cheese & Hazelnut Dip** 102

157 **Savory Lentil Dip** 102

158 **Mediterranean Trail Mix** 102

159 **Marinated Feta and Artichokes** 103

160 **Air Fryer Popcorn with Garlic Salt** 103

161 **Baked Spanakopita Dip** 103

162 **No-Mayo Tuna Salad Cucumber Bites** 104

163 **Goat Cheese–Mackerel Pâté** 104

164 **Burrata Caprese Stack** 104

165 **Baked Italian Spinach and Ricotta Balls** 105

166 **Steamed Artichokes with Herbs and Olive Oil** 105

167 **Fried Baby Artichokes with Lemon-Garlic Aioli** 106

168 **Shrimp and Chickpea Fritters** 106

169 **Crispy Spiced Chickpeas** 107

170 **Roasted Rosemary Olives** 107

171 **Artichoke and Olive Pita Flatbread** 107

172 **Roasted Pearl Onion Dip** 108

173 **Lemony Olives and Feta Medley** 108

174 **Cheese-Stuffed Dates** 108

175 **Sardine and Herb Bruschetta** 109

176 **Bravas-Style Potatoes** 109

Goat'S Cheese & Hazelnut Dip

Prep time: 10 minutes | Cook time: 0 minutes | Serves 8

2 heads (250 g/8.8 ounces) yellow chicory or endive
Pinch of salt
Dip
12 ounces (340 g) soft goat's cheese
1 tablespoon (15 ml) fresh lemon juice
1 clove garlic, minced
Salt, if needed, to taste
Topping
2 tablespoons (6 g/0.2 ounces) chopped fresh chives
1 tablespoon (15 ml) extra-virgin olive oil
Chile flakes or black pepper, to taste
Enough ice water to cover the leaves

3 tablespoons (45 ml) extra-virgin olive oil
1 teaspoon lemon zest (about ½ lemon)
Freshly ground black pepper, to taste

¼ cup (28 g/1 ounces) crushed hazelnuts, pecans, or walnuts

1. Cut off the bottom of the chicory and trim the leaves to get rid of any that are limp or brown. Place the leaves in salted ice water for 10 minutes. This will help the chicory leaves to become crisp. Drain and leave in the strainer.
2. To make the dip: Place the dip ingredients in a bowl and use a fork or spatula to mix until smooth and creamy. 3. Stir in the chives. Transfer to a serving bowl and top with the crushed hazelnuts, olive oil, and chile flakes. Serve with the crisp chicory leaves. Store in a sealed jar in the fridge for up to 5 days.

Per Serving
Total carbs: 2.1 g | Fiber: 1.5 g | Net Carbs: 0.6 g | Protein: 8.9 g | Fat: 18 g (of which saturated: 7.3 g) | Calories: 202

Savory Lentil Dip

Prep time: 10 minutes | Cook time: 32 minutes | Serves 16

2 tablespoons olive oil
3 cloves garlic, peeled and minced
4 cups water
¼ teaspoon ground black pepper

½ medium yellow onion, peeled and diced
2 cups dried red lentils, rinsed and drained
1 teaspoon salt
2 tablespoons minced fresh flat-leaf parsley

1. Press the Sauté button on the Instant Pot® and heat oil. Add onion and cook 2–3 minutes, or until translucent. Add garlic and cook until fragrant, about 30 seconds. Add lentils, water, and salt to pot, and stir to combine. Close lid, set steam release to Sealing, press the Bean button, and cook for the default time of 30 minutes. 2. When the timer beeps, let pressure release naturally for 10 minutes. Quick-release any remaining pressure until the float valve drops, then open lid. Transfer lentil mixture to a food processor and blend until smooth. Season with pepper and garnish with parsley. Serve warm.

Per Serving
Calories: 76 | Fat: 2g | Protein: 5g | Sodium: 145mg | Fiber: 2g | Carbohydrates: 11g | Sugar: 1g

Mediterranean Trail Mix

Prep time: 5 minutes | Cook time: 0 minutes | Serves 6

1 cup roughly chopped unsalted walnuts
½ cup shelled salted pistachios
½ cup roughly chopped dates

½ cup roughly chopped salted almonds
½ cup roughly chopped apricots
⅓ cup dried figs, sliced in half

1. In a large zip-top bag, combine the walnuts, almonds, pistachios, apricots, dates, and figs and mix well.

Per Serving
Calories: 348 | Protein: 9g | Total Carbohydrates: 33g | Sugars: 22g | Fiber: 7g | Total Fat: 24g | Saturated Fat: 2g | Cholesterol: 0mg | Sodium: 95mg

Marinated Feta and Artichokes

Prep time: 10 minutes | Cook time: 0 minutes | Makes 1½ cups

4 ounces (113 g) traditional Greek feta, cut into ½-inch cubes
⅓ cup extra-virgin olive oil
2 tablespoons roughly chopped fresh rosemary
½ teaspoon black peppercorns
4 ounces (113 g) drained artichoke hearts, quartered lengthwise
Zest and juice of 1 lemon
2 tablespoons roughly chopped fresh parsley

1. In a glass bowl or large glass jar, combine the feta and artichoke hearts. Add the olive oil, lemon zest and juice, rosemary, parsley, and peppercorns and toss gently to coat, being sure not to crumble the feta. 2. Cover and refrigerate for at least 4 hours, or up to 4 days. Pull out of the refrigerator 30 minutes before serving.

Per Serving
Calories: 235 | Total Fat: 23g | Total Carbs: 3g | Net Carbs: 2g | Fiber: 1g | Protein: 4g | Sodium: 406mg

Air Fryer Popcorn with Garlic Salt

Prep time: 3 minutes | Cook time: 10 minutes | Serves 2

2 tablespoons olive oil
1 teaspoon garlic salt
¼ cup popcorn kernels

1. Preheat the air fryer to 380ºF (193ºC). 2. Tear a square of aluminum foil the size of the bottom of the air fryer and place into the air fryer. 3. Drizzle olive oil over the top of the foil, and then pour in the popcorn kernels. 4. Roast for 8 to 10 minutes, or until the popcorn stops popping. 5. Transfer the popcorn to a large bowl and sprinkle with garlic salt before serving.

Per Serving
Calories: 245 | Total Fat: 15g | Saturated Fat: 2g | Protein: 4g | Total Carbohydrates: 25g | Fiber: 5g | Sugar: 0g | Cholesterol: 0mg

Baked Spanakopita Dip

Prep time: 10 minutes | Cook time: 15 minutes | Serves 2

Olive oil cooking spray
2 tablespoons minced white onion
4 cups fresh spinach
4 ounces (113 g) feta cheese, divided
¼ teaspoon ground nutmeg
½ teaspoon salt
3 tablespoons olive oil, divided
2 garlic cloves, minced
4 ounces (113 g) cream cheese, softened
Zest of 1 lemon
1 teaspoon dried dill
Pita chips, carrot sticks, or sliced bread for serving (optional)

1. Preheat the air fryer to 360ºF (182ºC). Coat the inside of a 6-inch ramekin or baking dish with olive oil cooking spray. 2. In a large skillet over medium heat, heat 1 tablespoon of the olive oil. Add the onion, then cook for 1 minute. 3. Add in the garlic and cook, stirring for 1 minute more. 4. Reduce the heat to low and mix in the spinach and water. Let this cook for 2 to 3 minutes, or until the spinach has wilted. Remove the skillet from the heat. 5. In a medium bowl, combine the cream cheese, 2 ounces of the feta, and the remaining 2 tablespoons of olive oil, along with the lemon zest, nutmeg, dill, and salt. Mix until just combined. 6. Add the vegetables to the cheese base and stir until combined. 7. Pour the dip mixture into the prepared ramekin and top with the remaining 2 ounces of feta cheese. 8. Place the dip into the air fryer basket and cook for 10 minutes, or until heated through and bubbling. 9. Serve with pita chips, carrot sticks, or sliced bread.

Per Serving
Calories: 550 | Total Fat: 52g | Saturated Fat: 22g | Protein: 14g | Total Carbohydrates: 9g | Fiber: 2g | Sugar: 5g | Cholesterol: 113mg

No-Mayo Tuna Salad Cucumber Bites

Prep time: 5 minutes | Cook time: 0 minutes | Serves 3

- 1 (5ounces/140g) can water-packed tuna, drained
- ½ teaspoons extra virgin olive oil
- 1 tablespoon chopped fresh dill
- Pinch of coarse sea salt
- 1 medium cucumber, cut into 15 (¼-inch/.5cm) thick slices
- ⅓ cup full-fat Greek yogurt
- 1 tablespoon finely chopped spring onion (white parts only)
- ¼ teaspoons freshly ground black pepper
- 1 teaspoon red wine vinegar

1. In a medium bowl, combine the tuna, yogurt, olive oil, spring onion, dill, sea salt, and black pepper. Mix well. 2. Arrange the cucumber slices on a plate and sprinkle the vinegar over the slices. 3. Place 1 heaping teaspoon of the tuna salad on top of each cucumber slice 4. Serve promptly. Store the tuna salad mixture covered in the refrigerator for up to 1 day.

Per Serving
Calories: 80 | Total fat: 3g | Saturated fat: 1g | Carbohydrate: 13g | Protein: 1g

Goat Cheese–Mackerel Pâté

Prep time: 10 minutes | Cook time: 0 minutes | Serves 4

- 4 ounces (113 g) olive oil-packed wild-caught mackerel
- Zest and juice of 1 lemon
- 2 tablespoons chopped fresh arugula
- 2 teaspoons chopped capers
- Crackers, cucumber rounds, endive spears, or celery, for serving (optional)
- 2 ounces goat cheese
- 2 tablespoons chopped fresh parsley
- 1 tablespoon extra-virgin olive oil
- 1 to 2 teaspoons fresh horseradish (optional)

1. In a food processor, blender, or large bowl with immersion blender, combine the mackerel, goat cheese, lemon zest and juice, parsley, arugula, olive oil, capers, and horseradish (if using). Process or blend until smooth and creamy. 2. Serve with crackers, cucumber rounds, endive spears, or celery. 3. Store covered in the refrigerator for up to 1 week.

Per Serving
Calories: 118 | Total Fat: 8g | Total Carbs: 1g | Net Carbs: 1g | Fiber: 0g | Protein: 9g | Sodium: 196mg

Burrata Caprese Stack

Prep time: 5 minutes | Cook time: 0 minutes | Serves 4

- 1 large organic tomato, preferably heirloom
- ¼ teaspoon freshly ground black pepper
- 8 fresh basil leaves, thinly sliced
- 1 tablespoon red wine or balsamic vinegar
- ½ teaspoon salt
- 1 (4 ounces / 113 g) ball burrata cheese
- 2 tablespoons extra-virgin olive oil

1. Slice the tomato into 4 thick slices, removing any tough center core and sprinkle with salt and pepper. Place the tomatoes, seasoned-side up, on a plate. 2. On a separate rimmed plate, slice the burrata into 4 thick slices and place one slice on top of each tomato slice. Top each with one-quarter of the basil and pour any reserved burrata cream from the rimmed plate over top. 3. Drizzle with olive oil and vinegar and serve with a fork and knife.

Per Serving (1 stack)
Calories: 153 | Total Fat: 13g | Total Carbs: 2g | Net Carbs: 1g | Fiber: 1g | Protein: 7g | Sodium: 469mg

Baked Italian Spinach and Ricotta Balls

Prep time: 15 minutes | Cook time: 2 minutes | Serves 4

- 1½ tablespoons extra virgin olive oil
- 9 ounces (255g) fresh baby leaf spinach, washed
- 9 ounces (255g) ricotta, drained
- 2 tablespoons chopped fresh basil
- ¼ teaspoons plus a pinch of freshly ground black pepper, divided
- 1 egg
- 1 garlic clove
- 3 spring onions (white parts only), thinly sliced
- 1.75 ounces (50g) grated Parmesan cheese
- ¾ teaspoons salt, divided
- 4½ tablespoons plus ⅓ cup unseasoned breadcrumbs, divided

1. Preheat the oven to 400°F (204°C). Line a large baking pan with parchment paper 2. Add the olive oil and garlic clove to a large pan over medium heat. When the oil begins to shimmer, add the spinach and sauté, tossing continuously, until the spinach starts to wilt, then add the spring onions. Continue tossing and sautéing until most of the liquid has evaporated, about 6 minutes, then transfer the spinach and onion mixture to a colander to drain and cool for 10 minutes. 3. When the spinach mixture has cooled, discard the garlic clove and squeeze the spinach to remove as much of the liquid as possible. Transfer the spinach mixture to a cutting board and finely chop. 4. Combine the ricotta, Parmesan, basil, ½ teaspoon of the salt, and ¼ teaspoon of the black pepper in a large bowl. Use a fork to mash the ingredients together, then add the spinach and continue mixing until the ingredients are combined. Add 4½ tablespoons of the breadcrumbs and mix until all ingredients are well combined. 5. In a small bowl, whisk the egg with the remaining ¼ teaspoon salt and a pinch of the black pepper. Place the remaining ⅓ cup of breadcrumbs on a small plate. Scoop out 1 tablespoon of the spinach mixture and roll it into a smooth ball, then dip it in the egg mixture and then roll it in the breadcrumbs. Place the ball on the prepared baking pan and continue the process with the remaining spinach mixture. 6. Bake for 16–20 minutes or until the balls turn a light golden brown. Remove the balls from the oven and serve promptly. Store covered in the refrigerator for up to 1 day. (Reheat before serving.)

Per Serving

Calories: 243 | Total fat: 13g | Saturated fat: 8g | Carbohydrate: 16g | Protein: 16g

Steamed Artichokes with Herbs and Olive Oil

Prep time: 10 minutes | Cook time: 10 minutes | Serves 6

- 3 medium artichokes with stems cut off
- 1 cup water
- ⅓ cup extra-virgin olive oil
- ¼ teaspoon salt
- 1 teaspoon chopped fresh rosemary
- 1 teaspoon fresh thyme leaves
- 1 medium lemon, halved
- ¼ cup lemon juice
- 1 clove garlic, peeled and minced
- 1 teaspoon chopped fresh oregano
- 1 teaspoon chopped fresh flat-leaf parsley

1. Run artichokes under running water, making sure water runs between leaves to flush out any debris. Slice off top ⅓ of artichoke and pull away any tough outer leaves. Rub all cut surfaces with lemon. 2. Add water and lemon juice to the Instant Pot®, then add rack. Place artichokes upside down on rack. Close lid, set steam release to Sealing, press the Manual button, and set time to 10 minutes. When the timer beeps, let pressure release naturally, about 20 minutes. 3. Press the Cancel button and open lid. Remove artichokes, transfer to a cutting board, and slice in half. Place halves on a serving platter. 4. In a small bowl, combine oil, garlic, salt, oregano, rosemary, parsley, and thyme. Drizzle half of mixture over artichokes, then serve remaining mixture in a small bowl for dipping. Serve warm.

Per Serving

Calories: 137 | Fat: 13g | Protein: 2g | Sodium: 158mg | Fiber: 4 | Carbohydrates: 7g | Sugar: 1g

Fried Baby Artichokes with Lemon-Garlic Aioli

Prep time: 5 minutes | Cook time: 50 minutes | Serves 10

Artichokes
½ lemon
Kosher salt, to taste
1 egg
1 tablespoon fresh lemon juice
½ cup olive oil

15 baby artichokes
3 cups olive oil
Aioli
2 cloves garlic, chopped
½ teaspoon Dijon mustard
Kosher salt and ground black pepper, to taste

To make the artichokes:
1. Wash and drain the artichokes. With a paring knife, strip off the coarse outer leaves around the base and stalk, leaving the softer leaves on. Carefully peel the stalks and trim off all but 2' below the base. Slice off the top ½' of the artichokes. Cut each artichoke in half. Rub the cut surfaces with a lemon half to keep from browning. 2. In a medium saucepan fitted with a deep-fry thermometer over medium heat, warm the oil to about 280°F (138 °C). Working in batches, cook the artichokes in the hot oil until tender, about 15 minutes. Using a slotted spoon, remove and drain on a paper towel–lined plate. Repeat with all the artichoke halves. 3. Increase the heat of the oil to 375°F (191°C). In batches, cook the precooked baby artichokes until browned at the edges and crisp, about 1 minute. Transfer to a paper towel–lined plate. Season with the salt to taste. Repeat with the remaining artichokes.

To make the aioli:
1. In a blender, pulse together the egg, garlic, lemon juice, and mustard until combined. With the blender running, slowly drizzle in the oil a few drops at a time until the mixture thickens like mayonnaise, about 2 minutes. Transfer to a bowl and season to taste with the salt and pepper. 2. Serve the warm artichokes with the aioli on the side.

Per Serving
Calories: 236 | Protein: 6g | Carbohydrates: 21g | Sugars: 2g | Total Fat: 17g | Saturated Fat: 3g | Fiber: 10g | Sodium: 283mg

Shrimp and Chickpea Fritters

Prep time: 5 minutes | Cook time: 10 minutes | Serves 6

2 tablespoons olive oil, plus ¼ cup, divided
12 ounces raw medium shrimp, peeled, deveined, and finely chopped
2 tablespoons roughly chopped parsley
½ teaspoon hot or sweet paprika
½ lemon

½ small yellow onion, finely chopped
¼ cup chickpea flour
2 tablespoon all-purpose flour
1 teaspoon baking powder
¾ teaspoon salt, plus additional to sprinkle over finished dish

1. Heat 2 tablespoons of the olive oil in a large skillet over medium-high heat. Add the onion and cook, stirring frequently, until softened, about 5 minutes. Using a slotted spoon, transfer the cooked onions to a medium bowl. Add the shrimp, chickpea flour, all-purpose flour, parsley, baking powder, paprika, and salt and mix well. Let sit for 10 minutes. 2. Heat the remaining ¼ cup olive oil in the same skillet set over medium-high heat. When the oil is very hot, add the batter, about 2 tablespoons at a time. Cook for about 2 minutes, until the bottom turns golden and the edges are crisp. Flip over and cook for another minute or two until the second side is golden and crisp. Drain on paper towels. Serve hot, with lemon squeezed over the top. Season with salt just before serving.

Per Serving
Calories: 148 | Total Fat: 6g | Saturated Fat: 1g | Carbs: 9g | Protein: 15g | Sodium: 435mg | Fiber: 3g

Crispy Spiced Chickpeas

Prep time: 5 minutes | Cook time: 25 minutes | Serves 6

3 cans (15 ounces / 425-g each) chickpeas, drained and rinsed
½ teaspoon ground cumin
¼ teaspoon ground cinnamon
1 cup olive oil
1 teaspoon paprika
½ teaspoon kosher salt
¼ teaspoon ground black pepper

1. Spread the chickpeas on paper towels and pat dry. 2. In a large saucepan over medium-high heat, warm the oil until shimmering. Add 1 chickpea | if it sizzles right away, the oil is hot enough to proceed. 3. Add enough chickpeas to form a single layer in the saucepan. Cook, occasionally gently shaking the saucepan until golden brown, about 8 minutes. With a slotted spoon, transfer to a paper towel–lined plate to drain. Repeat with the remaining chickpeas until all the chickpeas are fried. Transfer to a large bowl. 4. In a small bowl, combine the paprika, cumin, salt, cinnamon, and pepper. Sprinkle all over the fried chickpeas and toss to coat. The chickpeas will crisp as they cool.

Per Serving
Calories:175 | Protein: 6g | Carbohydrates: 20g | Sugars: 2g | Total Fat: 9g | Saturated Fat: 1g | Fiber: 5g | Sodium: 506mg

Roasted Rosemary Olives

Prep time: 5 minutes | Cook time: 25 minutes | Serves 4

1 cup mixed variety olives, pitted and rinsed
1 tablespoon extra-virgin olive oil
4 rosemary sprigs
2 tablespoons lemon juice
6 garlic cloves, peeled

1. Preheat the oven to 400°F (204°C). Line the baking sheet with parchment paper or foil. 2. Combine the olives, lemon juice, olive oil, and garlic in a medium bowl and mix together. Spread in a single layer on the prepared baking sheet. Sprinkle on the rosemary. Roast for 25 minutes, tossing halfway through. 3. Remove the rosemary leaves from the stem and place in a serving bowl. Add the olives and mix before serving.

Per Serving
Calories: 100 | Fat: 9g | Protein: 0g | Carbs: 4g | Sugars: 0g | Fiber: 0g | Sodium: 260mg | Cholesterol: 0mg

Artichoke and Olive Pita Flatbread

Prep time: 5 minutes | Cook time: 10 minutes | Serves 4

2 whole wheat pitas
2 garlic cloves, minced
½ cup canned artichoke hearts, sliced
¼ cup shredded Parmesan
Chopped fresh parsley, for garnish (optional)
2 tablespoons olive oil, divided
¼ teaspoon salt
¼ cup Kalamata olives
¼ cup crumbled feta

1. Preheat the air fryer to 380°F (193°C). 2. Brush each pita with 1 tablespoon olive oil, then sprinkle the minced garlic and salt over the top. 3. Distribute the artichoke hearts, olives, and cheeses evenly between the two pitas, and place both into the air fryer to bake for 10 minutes. 4. Remove the pitas and cut them into 4 pieces each before serving. Sprinkle parsley over the top, if desired.

Per Serving
Calories: 243 | Total Fat: 15g | Saturated Fat: 4g | Protein: 7g | Total Carbohydrates: 22g | Fiber: 5g | Sugar: 1g | Cholesterol: 12mg

Roasted Pearl Onion Dip

Prep time: 5 minutes | Cook time: 12 minutes | Serves 4

2 cups peeled pearl onions
3 tablespoons olive oil, divided
1 cup nonfat plain Greek yogurt
¼ teaspoon black pepper
Pita chips, vegetables, or toasted bread for serving (optional)

3 garlic cloves
½ teaspoon salt
1 tablespoon lemon juice
⅛ teaspoon red pepper flakes

1. Preheat the air fryer to 360°F (182°C). 2. In a large bowl, combine the pearl onions and garlic with 2 tablespoons of the olive oil until the onions are well coated. 3. Pour the garlic-and-onion mixture into the air fryer basket and roast for 12 minutes. 4. Transfer the garlic and onions to a food processor. Pulse the vegetables several times, until the onions are minced but still have some chunks. 5. In a large bowl, combine the garlic and onions and the remaining 1 tablespoon of olive oil, along with the salt, yogurt, lemon juice, black pepper, and red pepper flakes. 6. Cover and chill for 1 hour before serving with pita chips, vegetables, or toasted bread.

Per Serving
Calories: 150 | Total Fat: 10g | Saturated Fat: 1g | Protein: 7g | Total Carbohydrates: 8g | Fiber: 1g | Sugar: 4g | Cholesterol: 3mg

Lemony Olives and Feta Medley

Prep time: 10 minutes | Cook time: 0 minutes | Serves 8

1 (1-pound) block of Greek feta cheese
¼ cup extra-virgin olive oil
3 tablespoons lemon juice
1 teaspoon dried oregano

3 cups mixed olives (Kalamata and green), drained from brine; pitted preferred
1 teaspoon grated lemon zest
Pita bread, for serving

1. Cut the feta cheese into ½-inch squares and put them into a large bowl. 2. Add the olives to the feta and set aside. 3. In a small bowl, whisk together the olive oil, lemon juice, lemon zest, and oregano. 4. Pour the dressing over the feta cheese and olives and gently toss together to evenly coat everything. 5. Serve with pita bread.

Per Serving
Calories: 406 | Protein: 8g | Total Carbohydrates: 8g | Sugars: 2g | Fiber: 0g | Total Fat: 38g | Saturated Fat: 12g | Cholesterol: 51mg | Sodium: 1,658mg

Cheese-Stuffed Dates

Prep time: 10 minutes | Cook time: 10 minutes | Serves 4

2 ounces low-fat cream cheese, at room temperature
1 tablespoon low-fat plain Greek yogurt
¼ teaspoon kosher salt
Dash of hot sauce
8 medjool dates, pitted and halved

2 tablespoons sweet pickle relish
1 teaspoon finely chopped fresh chives
⅛ teaspoon ground black pepper
2 tablespoons pistachios, chopped

1. In a small bowl, stir together the cream cheese, relish, yogurt, chives, salt, pepper, and hot sauce. 2. Put the pistachios on a clean plate. Put the cream cheese mixture into a resealable plastic bag, and snip off 1 corner of the bag. Pipe the cream cheese mixture into the date halves and press the tops into the pistachios to coat.

Per Serving
Calories:196 | Protein: 3g | Carbohydrates: 41g | Sugars: 35g | Total Fat: 4g | Saturated Fat: 1.5g | Fiber: 4g | Sodium: 294mg

Sardine and Herb Bruschetta

Prep time: 5 minutes | Cook time: 10 minutes | Serves 4

8 (1-inch/2.5cm) thick whole-grain baguette slices
4 ounces (115g) olive oil–packed sardines (about 1 can)
2 tablespoons capers, drained
½ teaspoons dried oregano
1 garlic clove, halved
1½ tablespoons extra virgin olive oil
2 tablespoons fresh lemon juice
1 teaspoon red wine vinegar
3 tablespoons finely chopped onion (any variety)
1 tablespoon finely chopped fresh mint

1. Preheat the oven to 400°F (204°C). 2. Place the baguette slices on a large baking sheet and brush them with the olive oil. Transfer to the oven and toast until the slices are golden, about 10 minutes. 3. While the baguette slices are toasting, make the sardine topping by combining the sardines, lemon juice, and vinegar in a medium bowl. Mash with a fork. Add the capers, onions, oregano, and mint, and stir to combine. 4. When the baguette slices are done toasting, remove them from the oven and rub them with the garlic. 5. Transfer the slices to a serving platter. Place 1 heaping tablespoon of the topping onto each baguette slice. Store the sardine topping in the refrigerator for up to 3 days.

Per Serving
Calories: 193 | Total fat: 9g | Saturated fat: 1g | Carbohydrate: 16g | Protein: 11g

Bravas-Style Potatoes

Prep time: 15 minutes | Cook time: 50 minutes | Serves 8

4 large russet potatoes (about 2½ pounds), scrubbed and cut into 1' cubes
½ teaspoon ground black pepper
½ small yellow onion, chopped
1 tablespoon sherry vinegar
1 tablespoon chopped fresh flat-leaf parsley
Hot sauce (optional)
4 teaspoons olive oil, divided
1 teaspoon kosher salt, divided
¼ teaspoon red-pepper flakes
1 large tomato, chopped
1 teaspoon hot paprika

1. Preheat the oven to 450°F (235°C). Bring a large pot of well-salted water to a boil. 2. Boil the potatoes until just barely tender, 5 to 8 minutes. Drain and transfer the potatoes to a large rimmed baking sheet. Add 1 tablespoon of the oil, ½ teaspoon of the salt, the black pepper, and pepper flakes. With 2 large spoons, toss very well to coat the potatoes in the oil. Spread the potatoes out on the baking sheet. Roast until the bottoms are starting to brown and crisp, 20 minutes. Carefully flip the potatoes and roast until the other side is golden and crisp, 15 to 20 minutes. 3. Meanwhile, in a small skillet over medium heat, warm the remaining 1 teaspoon oil. Cook the onion until softened, 3 to 4 minutes. Add the tomato and cook until it's broken down and saucy, 5 minutes. Stir in the vinegar, paprika, and the remaining ½ teaspoon salt. Cook for 30 seconds, remove from the heat, and cover to keep warm. 4. Transfer the potatoes to a large serving bowl. Drizzle the tomato mixture over the potatoes. Sprinkle with the parsley. Serve with hot sauce, if using.

Per Serving
Calories: 173 | Protein: 4g | Carbohydrates: 35g | Sugars: 2g | Total Fat: 2g | Saturated Fat: 0.5g | Fiber: 3g | Sodium: 251mg

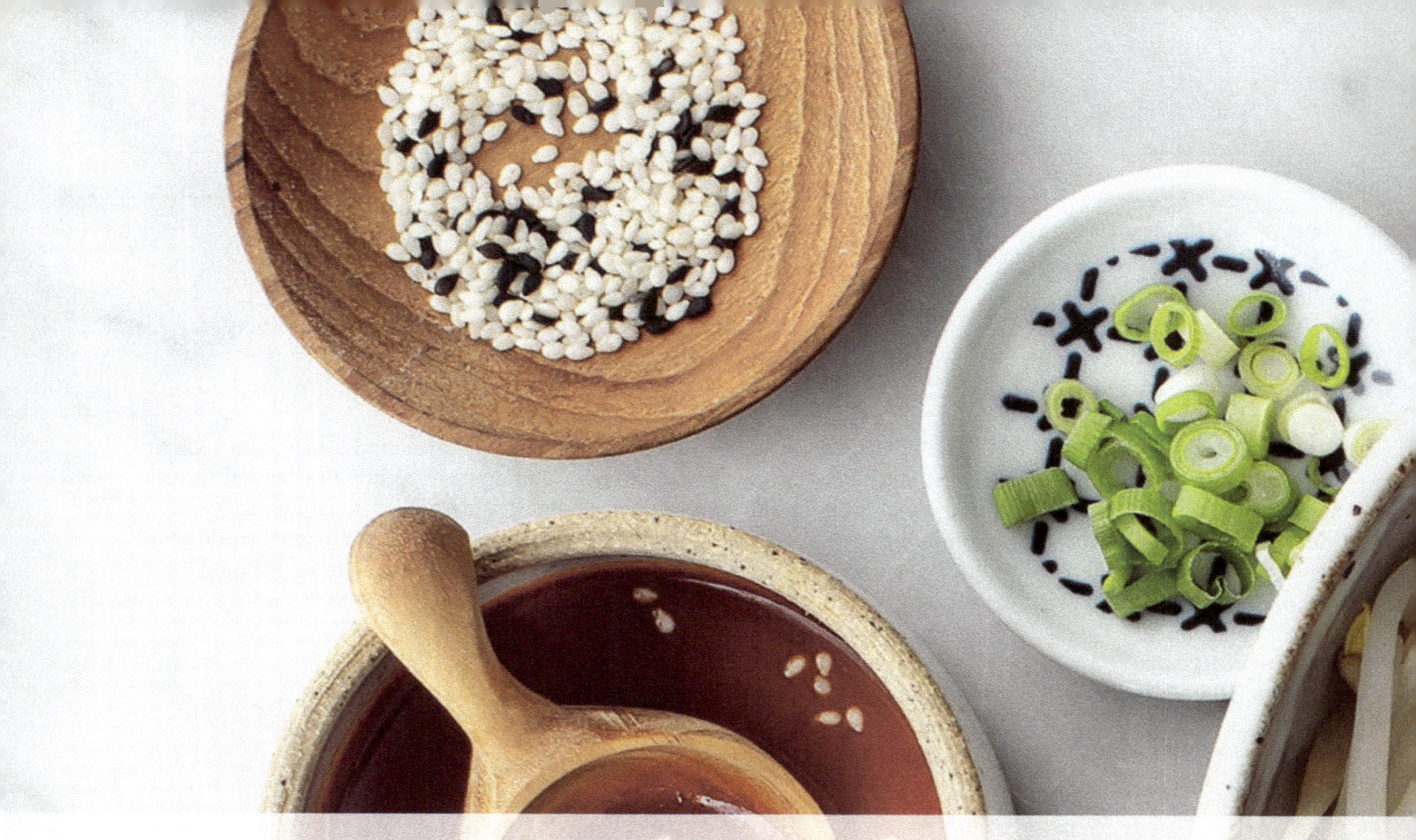

Chapter 12 Staples, Sauces, Dips, and Dressings

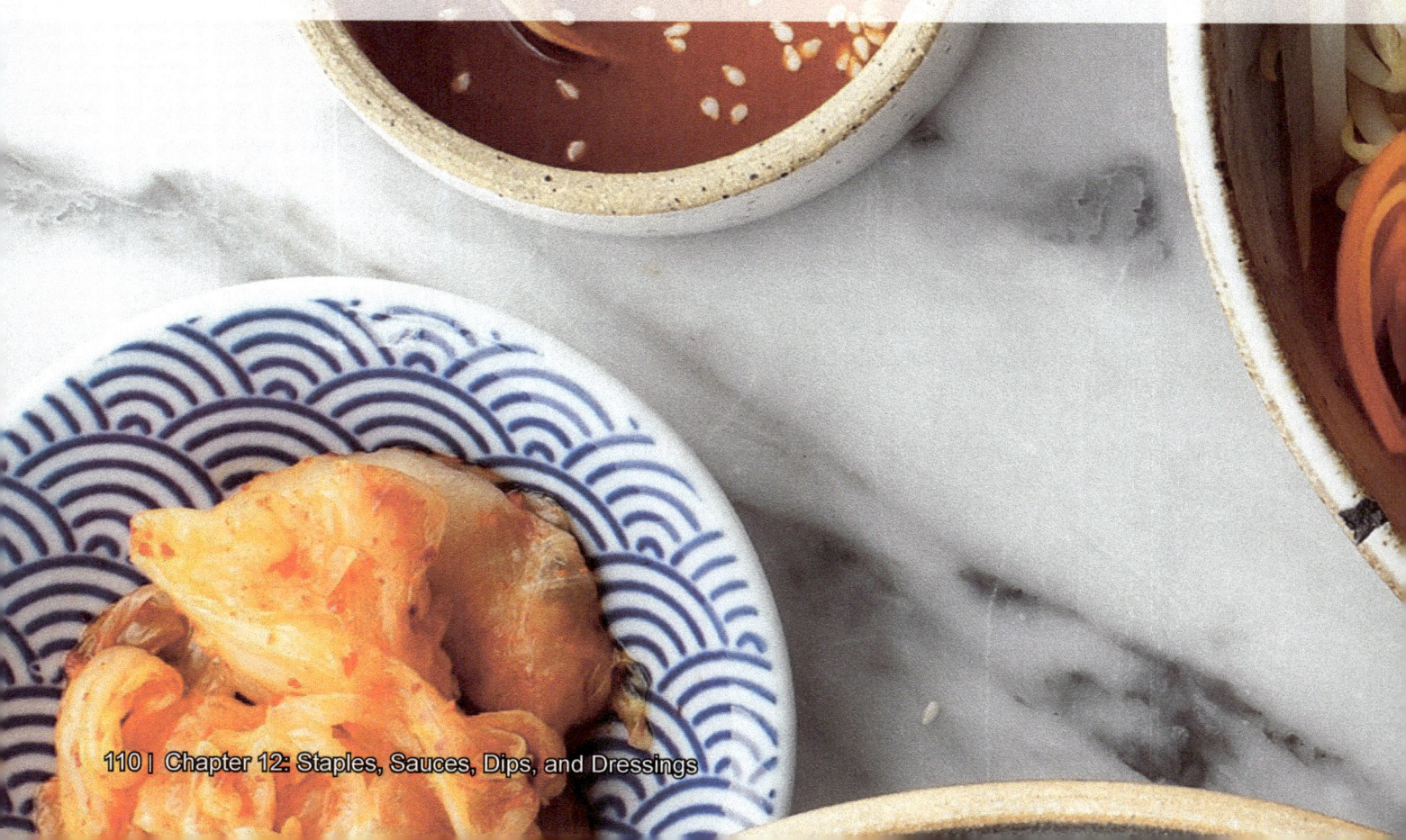

177	**Roasted Harissa**	**112**
178	**Kidney Bean Dip with Cilantro, Cumin, and Lime**	**112**
179	**Lemon Tahini Dressing**	**112**
180	**Red Pepper Chimichurri**	**113**
181	**Vinaigrette**	**113**
182	**Sherry Vinaigrette**	**113**
183	**Citrus Vinaigrette**	**113**
184	**Red Pepper Hummus**	**114**
185	**Zucchini Noodles**	**114**
186	**Melitzanosalata (Greek Eggplant Dip)**	**114**
187	**Skinny Cider Dressing**	**115**
188	**Tabil (Tunisian Five-Spice Blend)**	**115**
189	**Dijon Vinaigrette**	**115**
190	**Green Olive Tapenade with Harissa**	**115**
191	**Riced Cauliflower**	**116**

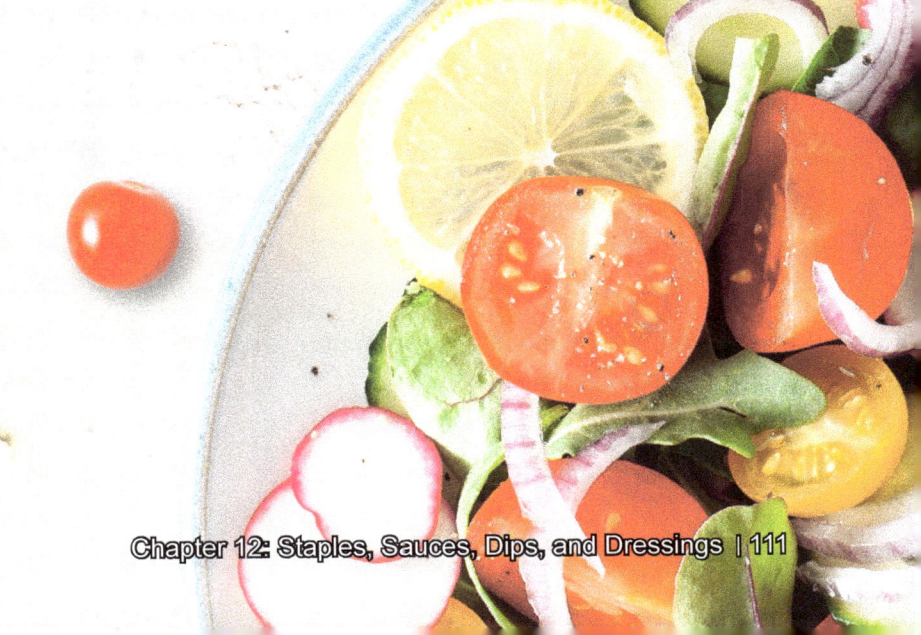

Roasted Harissa

Prep time: 5 minutes | Cook time: 15 minutes | Makes ¾ cup

- 1 red bell pepper
- 4 garlic cloves, unpeeled
- ½ teaspoon ground cumin
- 1 tablespoon fresh lemon juice
- 2 small fresh red chiles, or more to taste
- ½ teaspoon ground coriander
- ½ teaspoon ground caraway
- ½ teaspoon salt

1. Preheat the broiler to high. 2. Put the bell pepper, chiles, and garlic on a baking sheet and broil for 6 to 8 minutes. Turn the vegetables over and broil for 5 to 6 minutes more, until the pepper and chiles are softened and blackened. Remove from the broiler and set aside until cool enough to handle. Remove and discard the stems, skin, and seeds from the pepper and chiles. Remove and discard the papery skin from the garlic. 3. Put the flesh of the pepper and chiles with the garlic cloves in a blender or food processor. Add the coriander, cumin, caraway, lemon juice, and salt and blend until smooth. 4. This may be stored refrigerated for up to 3 days. Store in an airtight container, and cover the sauce with a ¼-inch layer of oil.

Per Serving
Calories: 28 | Fat: 0g | Protein: 1g | Carbs: 6g | Sugars: 3g | Fiber: 1g | Sodium: 393mg | Cholesterol: 0mg

Kidney Bean Dip with Cilantro, Cumin, and Lime

Prep time: 10 minutes | Cook time: 30 minutes | Serves 16

- 1 cup dried kidney beans, soaked overnight and drained
- 3 cloves garlic, peeled and crushed
- ¼ cup extra-virgin olive oil
- 2 teaspoons grated lime zest
- ½ teaspoon salt
- 4 cups water
- ¼ cup roughly chopped cilantro, divided
- 1 tablespoon lime juice
- 1 teaspoon ground cumin

1. Place beans, water, garlic, and 2 tablespoons cilantro in the Instant Pot®. Close the lid, set steam release to Sealing, press the Bean button, and cook for the default time of 30 minutes. 2. When the timer beeps, let pressure release naturally, about 20 minutes. Press the Cancel button, open lid, and check that beans are tender. Drain off excess water and transfer beans to a medium bowl. Gently mash beans with potato masher or fork until beans are mashed but chunky. Add oil, lime juice, lime zest, cumin, salt, and remaining 2 tablespoons cilantro and stir to combine. Serve warm or at room temperature.

Per Serving
Calories: 65 | Fat: 3g | Protein: 2g | Sodium: 75mg | Fiber: 2 | Carbohydrates: 7g | Sugar: 0g

Lemon Tahini Dressing

Prep time: 5 minutes | Cook time: 0 minutes | Makes ½ cup

- ¼ cup tahini
- 3 tablespoons warm water
- ¼ teaspoon pure maple syrup
- ⅛ teaspoon cayenne pepper
- 3 tablespoons lemon juice
- ¼ teaspoon kosher salt
- ¼ teaspoon ground cumin

In a medium bowl, whisk together the tahini, lemon juice, water, salt, maple syrup, cumin, and cayenne pepper until smooth. Place in the refrigerator until ready to serve. Store any leftovers in the refrigerator in an airtight container up to 5 days.

Per Serving (2 tablespoons)
Calories: 90 | Fat: 7g | Protein: 3g | Carbs: 5g | Sugars: 1g | Fiber: 1g | Sodium: 80mg | Cholesterol: 0mg

Red Pepper Chimichurri

Prep time: 10 minutes | Cook time: 0 minutes | Serves 4

1 garlic clove, minced
1 tablespoon red wine vinegar or sherry vinegar
1 shallot, finely chopped
3 tablespoons capers, rinsed
3 tablespoons chopped fresh parsley
3 tablespoons olive oil
¼ teaspoon freshly ground black pepper
1 large red bell pepper, roasted, peeled, seeded, and finely chopped (about 1 cup)
½ teaspoon red pepper flakes

1. In a small bowl, stir together all the ingredients until well combined.

Per Serving
Calories: 113 | Fat: 10g | Protein: 1g | Carbs: 5g | Sugars: 2g | Fiber: 1g | Sodium: 157mg | Cholesterol: 0mg

Vinaigrette

Prep time: 5 minutes | Cook time: 0 minutes | Serves 4

2 tablespoons balsamic vinegar
1 teaspoon dried rosemary, crushed
¼ cup olive oil
2 large garlic cloves, minced
¼ teaspoon freshly ground black pepper

1. In a small bowl, whisk together the vinegar, garlic, rosemary, and pepper. While whisking, slowly stream in the olive oil and whisk until emulsified. Store in an airtight container in the refrigerator for up to 3 days.

Per Serving (1 cup)
Calories: 129 | Fat: 1g | Protein: 3g | Carbs: 0g | Sugars: 1g | Fiber: 0g | Sodium: 2mg | Cholesterol: 0mg

Sherry Vinaigrette

Prep time: 5 minutes | Cook time: 0 minutes | Makes about ¾ cup

⅓ cup sherry vinegar
2 teaspoons dried oregano
½ teaspoon freshly ground black pepper
1 clove garlic
1 teaspoon salt
½ cup olive oil

1. In a food processor or blender, combine the vinegar, garlic, oregano, salt, and pepper and process until the garlic is minced and the ingredients are well combined. With the food processor running, add the olive oil in a thin stream until it is well incorporated. Serve immediately or store, covered, in the refrigerator for up to a week.

Per Serving
Calories: 74 | Total Fat: 8g | Saturated Fat: 1g | Carbs: 0g | Protein: 0g | Sodium: 194mg | Fiber: 0g

Citrus Vinaigrette

Prep time: 2 minutes | Cook time: 0 minutes | Serves 4

Zest of 1 lemon
Pinch kosher salt
2 tablespoons olive oil
3 tablespoons fresh lemon juice
Pinch freshly ground black pepper

1. In a small bowl, whisk together the lemon zest, lemon juice, 3 tablespoons water, the salt, and the pepper. While whisking, gradually stream in the olive oil and whisk until emulsified. Store in an airtight container in the refrigerator for up to 3 days.

Per Serving
Calories: 65 | Fat: 7g | Protein: 0g | Carbs: 2g | Sugars: 1g | Fiber: 0g | Sodium: 146mg | Cholesterol: 0mg

Red Pepper Hummus

Prep time: 5 minutes | Cook time: 30 minutes | Makes 2 cups

1 cup dried chickpeas
1 tablespoon plus ¼ cup extra-virgin olive oil, divided
1 teaspoon ground cumin
½ teaspoon ground black pepper
⅓ cup lemon juice

4 cups water
½ cup chopped roasted red pepper, divided
⅓ cup tahini
¾ teaspoon salt
¼ teaspoon smoked paprika
½ teaspoon minced garlic

1. Place chickpeas, water, and 1 tablespoon oil in the Instant Pot®. Close the lid, set steam release to Sealing, press the Manual button, and set time to 30 minutes. 2. When the timer beeps, quick-release the pressure until the float valve drops. Press the Cancel button and open lid. Drain, reserving the cooking liquid. 3. Place chickpeas, ⅓ cup roasted red pepper, remaining ¼ cup oil, tahini, cumin, salt, black pepper, paprika, lemon juice, and garlic in a food processor and process until creamy. If hummus is too thick, add reserved cooking liquid 1 tablespoon at a time until it reaches desired consistency. Serve at room temperature, garnished with reserved roasted red pepper on top.

Per Serving (2 tablespoons)
Calories: 96 | Fat: 8g | Protein: 2g | Sodium: 122mg | Fiber: 4 | Carbohydrates: 10g | Sugar: 0g

Zucchini Noodles

Prep time: 5 minutes | Cook time: 0 minutes | Serves 4

2 medium to large zucchini

1. Cut off and discard the ends of each zucchini and, using a spiralizer set to the smallest setting, spiralize the zucchini to create zoodles. 2. To serve, simply place a ½ cup or so of spiralized zucchini into the bottom of each bowl and spoon a hot sauce over top to "cook" the zoodles to al dente consistency. Use with any of your favorite sauces, or just toss with warmed pesto for a simple and quick meal.

Per Serving
Calories: 48 | Total Fat: 1g | Total Carbs: 7g | Net Carbs: 4g | Fiber: 3g | Protein: 6g | Sodium: 7mg

Melitzanosalata (Greek Eggplant Dip)

Prep time: 10 minutes | Cook time: 3 minutes | Serves 8

1 cup water
1 clove garlic, peeled
1 tablespoon red wine vinegar
2 tablespoons minced fresh parsley

1 large eggplant, peeled and chopped
½ teaspoon salt
½ cup extra-virgin olive oil

1. Add water to the Instant Pot®, add the rack to the pot, and place the steamer basket on the rack. 2. Place eggplant in steamer basket. Close lid, set steam release to Sealing, press the Manual button, and set time to 3 minutes. When the timer beeps, quick-release the pressure until the float valve drops. Press the Cancel button and open lid. 3. Transfer eggplant to a food processor and add garlic, salt, and vinegar. Pulse until smooth, about 20 pulses. 4. Slowly add oil to the eggplant mixture while the food processor runs continuously until oil is completely incorporated. Stir in parsley. Serve at room temperature.

Per Serving
Calories: 134 | Fat: 14g | Protein: 1g | Sodium: 149mg | Fiber: 2 | Carbohydrates: 3g | Sugar: 2g

Skinny Cider Dressing

Prep time: 5 minutes | Cook time: 0 minutes | Serves 2

2 tablespoons apple cider vinegar
⅓ lemon, zested
Freshly ground black pepper
⅓ lemon, juiced
Salt

1. In a jar, combine the vinegar, lemon juice, and zest. Season with salt and pepper, cover, and shake well.

Per Serving
Calories: 2 | Protein: 0g | Total Carbohydrates: 1g | Sugars: 1g | Fiber: 1g | Total Fat: 0g | Saturated Fat: 0g | Cholesterol: 0mg | Sodium: 1mg

Tabil (Tunisian Five-Spice Blend)

Prep time: 2 minutes | Cook time: 0 minutes | Makes 2 tablespoons

1 tablespoon ground coriander
¼ teaspoon garlic powder
¼ teaspoon ground cumin
1 teaspoon caraway seeds
¼ teaspoon cayenne pepper

1. Combine all the ingredients in a small bowl. 2. It may be stored in an airtight container for up to 2 weeks.

Per Serving
Calories: 13 | Fat: 1g | Protein: 1g | Carbs: 2g | Sugars: 0g | Fiber: 1g | Sodium: 2mg | Cholesterol: 0mg

Dijon Vinaigrette

Prep time: 5 minutes | Cook time: 0 minutes | Serves 4

2 tablespoons Dijon mustard
1 garlic clove, finely minced
Pink Himalayan salt
3 tablespoons olive oil
Juice of ½ lemon
1½ tablespoons red wine vinegar
Freshly ground black pepper

1. In a small bowl, whisk the mustard, lemon juice, garlic, and red wine vinegar until well combined. Season with pink Himalayan salt and pepper, and whisk again. 2. Slowly add the olive oil, a little bit at a time, whisking constantly. 3. Keep in a sealed glass container in the refrigerator for up to 1 week.

Per Serving
Calories: 99 | Total Fat: 11g | Carbs: 1g | Net Carbs: 1g | Fiber: 1g | Protein: 1g

Green Olive Tapenade with Harissa

Prep time: 5 minutes | Cook time: 0 minutes | Makes about 1½ cups

1 cup pitted, cured green olives
1 tablespoon harissa
1 tablespoon chopped fresh parsley
1 clove garlic, minced
1 tablespoon lemon juice
¼ cup olive oil, or more to taste

1. Finely chop the olives (or pulse them in a food processor until they resemble a chunky paste). 2. Add the garlic, harissa, lemon juice, parsley, and olive oil and stir or pulse to combine well.

Per Serving
Calories: 215 | total fat: 23g | saturated fat: 3g | carbs: 5g | protein: 1g | sodium: 453mg | fiber: 2g

Riced Cauliflower

Prep time: 5 minutes | Cook time: 10 minutes | Serves 6 to 8

1 small head cauliflower, broken into florets
2 garlic cloves, finely minced
½ teaspoon freshly ground black pepper
¼ cup extra-virgin olive oil
1½ teaspoons salt

1. Place the florets in a food processor and pulse several times, until the cauliflower is the consistency of rice or couscous. 2. In a large skillet, heat the olive oil over medium-high heat. Add the cauliflower, garlic, salt, and pepper and sauté for 5 minutes, just to take the crunch out but not enough to let the cauliflower become soggy. 3. Remove the cauliflower from the skillet and place in a bowl until ready to use. Toss with chopped herbs and additional olive oil for a simple side, top with sautéed veggies and protein, or use in your favorite recipe.

Per Serving
Calories: 92 | Total Fat: 9g | Total Carbs: 3g | Net Carbs: 2g | Fiber: 1g | Protein: 1g | Sodium: 595mg

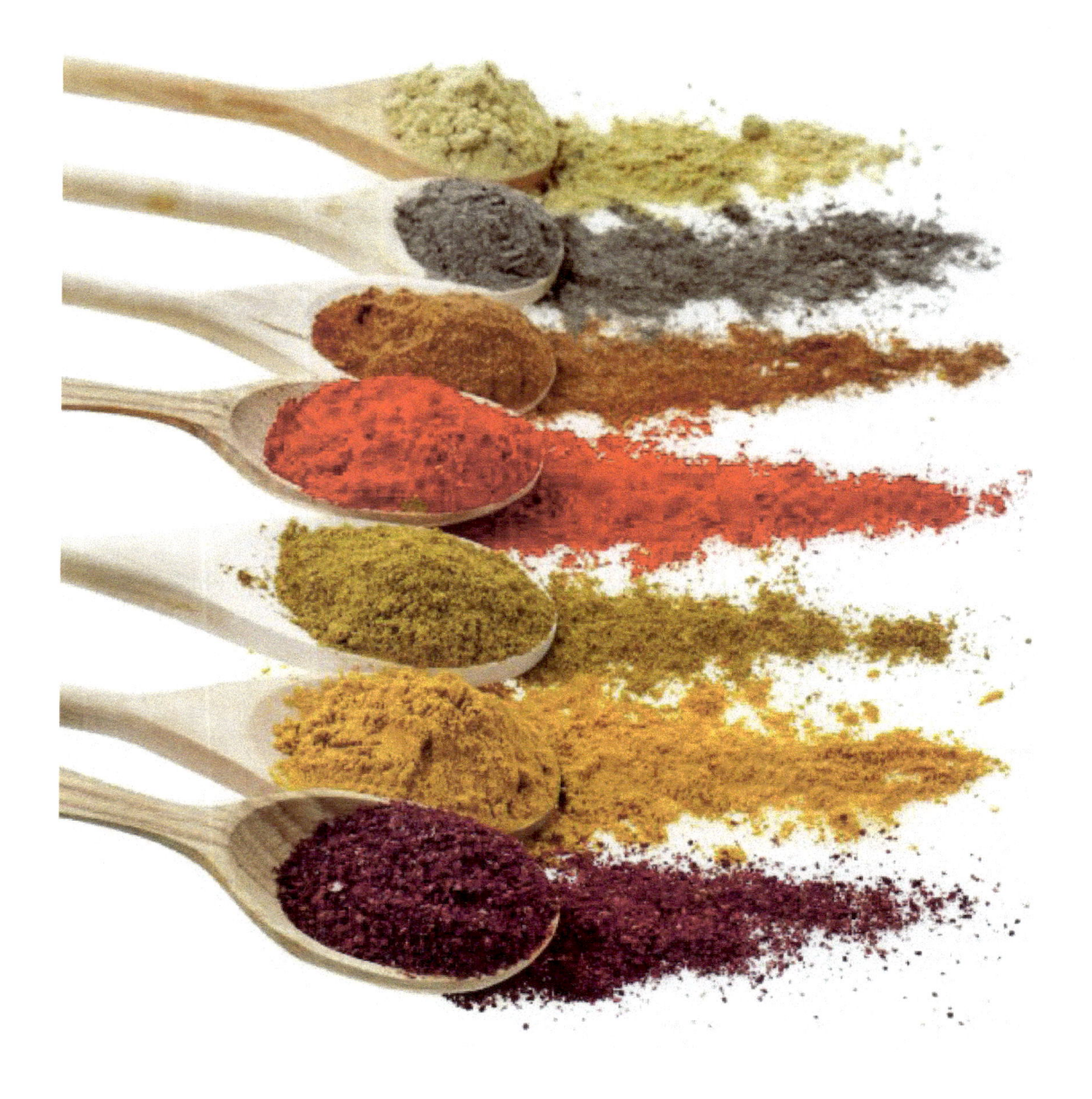

Chapter 13   Stews and Soups

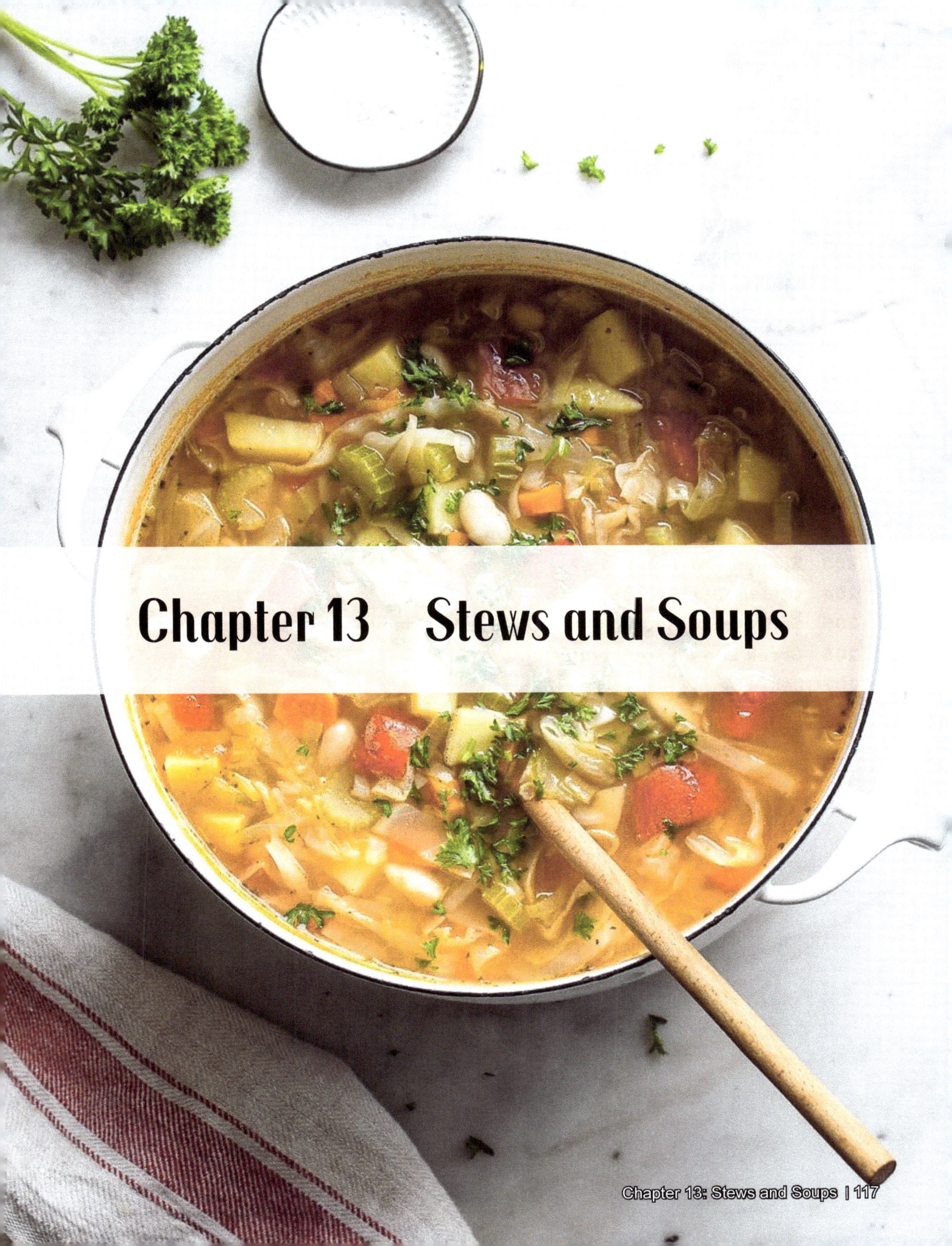

192	**Spanish-Style Turkey Meatball Soup**	119
193	**Spicy Sausage Lentil Soup**	119
194	**Mediterranean Vegetable Soup**	120
195	**Tunisian Bean Soup with Poached Eggs**	120
196	**Lemon Orzo Chicken Soup**	120
197	**Lentil and Chorizo Soup**	121
198	**Cream of Cauliflower Gazpacho**	121
199	**Lentil Sweet Potato Soup**	122
200	**Greek Salad Soup**	122
201	**Tuscan Bean Soup with Kale**	122
202	**Cauliflower & Blue Cheese Soup**	123
203	**Sicilian Fish Soup**	123
204	**Lemon Chicken Soup with Orzo**	124
205	**Saffron-Scented Chickpea Soup with Crispy Pasta**	124
206	**Greek Lemon Soup with Quinoa**	125
207	**Lentil Soup with Sorrel**	125

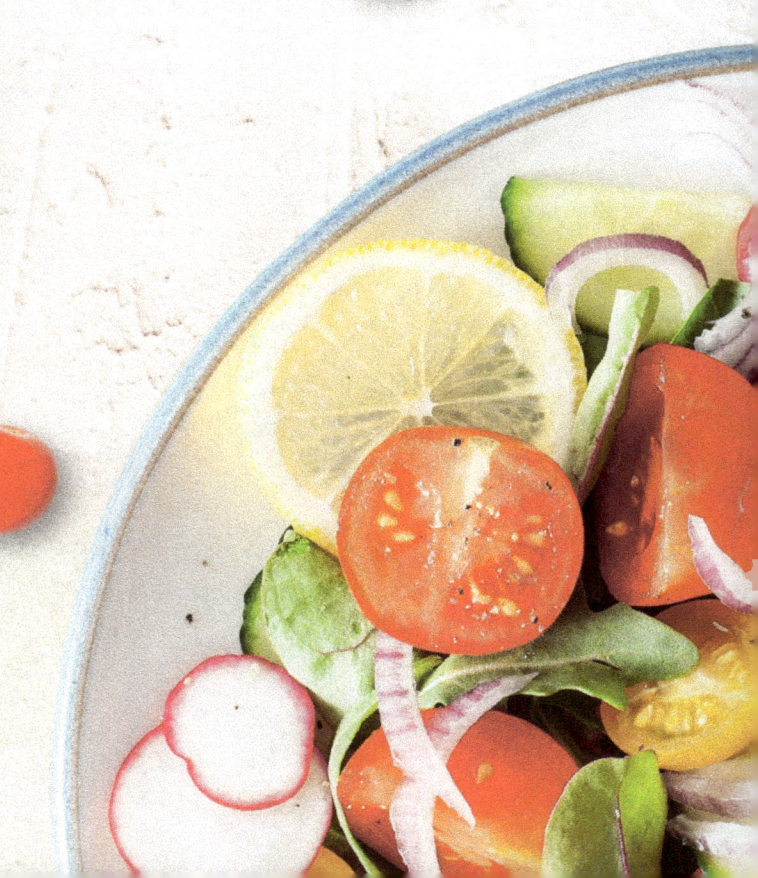

Spanish-Style Turkey Meatball Soup

Prep time: 10 minutes | Cook time: 15 minutes | Serves 6 to 8

1 slice hearty white sandwich bread, torn into quarters
1 ounce Manchego cheese, grated (½ cup), plus extra for serving
1 pound (454 g) ground turkey
1 onion, chopped
4 garlic cloves, minced
2 teaspoons smoked paprika
8 cups chicken broth
¼ cup whole milk
5 tablespoons minced fresh parsley, divided
½ teaspoon table salt
1 tablespoon extra-virgin olive oil
1 red bell pepper, stemmed, seeded, and cut into ¾-inch pieces
½ cup dry white wine
8 ounces (227 g) kale, stemmed and chopped

1. Using fork, mash bread and milk together into paste in large bowl. Stir in Manchego, 3 tablespoons parsley, and salt until combined. Add turkey and knead mixture with your hands until well combined. Pinch off and roll 2-teaspoon-size pieces of mixture into balls and arrange on large plate (you should have about 35 meatballs); set aside. 2. Using highest sauté function, heat oil in Instant Pot until shimmering. Add onion and bell pepper and cook until softened and lightly browned, 5 to 7 minutes. Stir in garlic and paprika and cook until fragrant, about 30 seconds. Stir in wine, scraping up any browned bits, and cook until almost completely evaporated, about 5 minutes. Stir in broth and kale, then gently submerge meatballs. 3. Lock lid in place and close pressure release valve. Select high pressure cook function and cook for 3 minutes. Turn off Instant Pot and quick-release pressure. Carefully remove lid, allowing steam to escape away from you. 4. Stir in remaining 2 tablespoons parsley and season with salt and pepper to taste. Serve, passing extra Manchego separately.

Per Serving
Cal: 170 | Total Fat: 4.5g | Sat Fat: 2.5g | Chol: 25mg | Sodium: 750mg | Total Carbs: 9g, Fiber: 2g, Total Sugar: 4g | Added Sugar: 0g | Protein: 21g

Spicy Sausage Lentil Soup

Prep timePrep Time: 30 minutes | Cook Time: 60 minutes | Serves 2

1 tablespoon olive oil
2 links (8 ounces / 227 g)) spicy Italian sausage (turkey or pork), removed from casing
2 garlic cloves, minced
½ teaspoon thyme
1 teaspoon oregano
3 cups low-sodium chicken stock
¾ cup brown lentils
½ teaspoon salt, plus more to taste
½ medium onion, diced (about ¾ cup)
2 medium carrots, sliced into coins (about ¾ cup)
1 medium celery stalk, diced (about ¼ cup)
¼ teaspoon red pepper flakes (omit or use less if you prefer less spicy)
1 bay leaf
1 (28 ounces / 794 g) can crushed tomatoes
1 cup packed baby spinach, sliced

1. Heat the oil in a stockpot over medium-high heat. Add the onion and sausage and sauté, breaking up the sausage into small pieces. 2. Add the carrots, celery, and garlic, and continue to sauté for about 10 more minutes. 3. Add the red pepper flakes, thyme, oregano, bay leaf, chicken stock, and tomatoes. Bring the soup to a boil. 4. Reduce the heat to medium-low and add the lentils. Stir everything well, cover, and let the soup simmer for 45 minutes, or until the lentils and carrots are tender. 5. Remove the bay leaf. Add the spinach and season with salt—start with ½ teaspoon and add additional salt to taste.

Per Serving
Calories: 354 | Total fat: 9g | Total carbs: 45g | Fiber: 12g | Sugar: 13g | Protein: 25g | Sodium: 694mg | Cholesterol: 17mg

Mediterranean Vegetable Soup

Prep time: 20 minutes | Cook time: 6 to 8 hours | Serves 6

1 (28 ounces / 794 g) can no-salt-added diced tomatoes
1 green bell pepper, seeded and chopped
4 ounces (113 g) mushrooms, sliced
1 small red onion, chopped
1 tablespoon extra-virgin olive oil
1 teaspoon paprika
½ teaspoon freshly ground black pepper
2 cups low-sodium vegetable broth
1 red or yellow bell pepper, seeded and chopped
2 zucchini, chopped
3 garlic cloves, minced
2 teaspoons dried oregano
1 teaspoon sea salt
Juice of 1 lemon

1. In a slow cooker, combine the tomatoes, vegetable broth, green and red bell peppers, mushrooms, zucchini, onion, garlic, olive oil, oregano, paprika, salt, and black pepper. Stir to mix well. 2. Cover the cooker and cook for 6 to 8 hours on Low heat. 3. Stir in the lemon juice before serving.

Per Serving
Calories: 91 | Total fat: 3g | Sodium: 502mg | Carbohydrates: 16g | Fiber: 5g | Sugar: 9g | Protein: 3g

Tunisian Bean Soup with Poached Eggs

Prep time: 10 minutes | Cook time: 25 minutes | Serves 4

2 tablespoons olive oil
1 carrot, finely chopped
3 tablespoons harissa
1 (15 ounces / 425-g) can chickpeas, drained
4 eggs
1 small red onion, finely chopped
4 garlic cloves, minced
3 cups vegetable broth
1 (5 ounces / 142-g) bag watercress or baby spinach (or red cabbage)

1. In a large saucepan, heat the olive oil over medium heat. Add the onion, carrot, garlic, and harissa. Cook until the vegetables are softened, 10 to 12 minutes. 2. Add the broth, chickpeas, and greens. Cook for 8 to 10 minutes, until the greens are cooked. Carefully add the eggs to the soup, one at a time. Cover; poach the eggs in the soup to your desired doneness, about 5 minutes. 3. Ladle the soup into bowls, top each with 1 egg, and serve.

Per Serving (1 cup)
Calories: 373 | Fat: 20g | Protein: 18g | Carbs: 32g | Sugars: 8g | Fiber: 8g | Sodium: 583mg | Cholesterol: 579mg

Lemon Orzo Chicken Soup

Prep time: 10 minutes | Cook time: 20 minutes | Serves 8

1 tablespoon extra-virgin olive oil
½ cup chopped carrots
3 garlic cloves, minced
2 cups shredded cooked chicken breast
Zest of 1 lemon, grated
8 ounces (227 g) cooked orzo pasta
1 cup chopped onion
½ cup chopped celery
9 cups low-sodium chicken broth
½ cup freshly squeezed lemon juice
1 to 2 teaspoons dried oregano

1. In a large pot, heat the oil over medium heat and add the onion, carrots, celery, and garlic and cook for about 5 minutes, until the onions are translucent. Add the broth and bring to a boil. 2. Reduce to a simmer, cover, and cook for 10 more minutes, until the flavors meld. Then add the shredded chicken, lemon juice and zest, and oregano. 3. Plate the orzo in serving bowls first, then add the chicken soup.

Per Serving
Calories: 215 | Protein: 16g | Total Carbohydrates: 27g | Sugars: 2g | Fiber: 2g | Total Fat: 5g | Saturated Fat: 1g | Cholesterol: 26mg | Sodium: 114mg

Lentil and Chorizo Soup

Prep time: 25 minutes | Cook time: 20 minutes | Serves 6 to 8

- 1 tablespoon extra-virgin olive oil, plus extra for drizzling
- 4 garlic cloves, minced
- 5 cups water
- 4 cups chicken broth
- 1 tablespoon sherry vinegar, plus extra for seasoning
- 1 teaspoon table salt
- 2 carrots, peeled and halved crosswise
- ½ cup minced fresh parsley
- 8 ounces (227 g) Spanish-style chorizo sausage, quartered lengthwise and sliced thin
- 1½ teaspoons smoked paprika
- 1 pound (454 g) (2¼ cups) French green lentils, picked over and rinsed
- 2 bay leaves
- 1 large onion, peeled
- ½ cup slivered almonds, toasted

1. Using highest sauté function, heat oil in Instant Pot until shimmering. Add chorizo and cook until lightly browned, 3 to 5 minutes. Stir in garlic and paprika and cook until fragrant, about 30 seconds. Stir in water, scraping up any browned bits, then stir in lentils, broth, vinegar, bay leaves, and salt. Nestle onion and carrots into pot. 2. Lock lid in place and close pressure release valve. Select high pressure cook function and cook for 14 minutes. Turn off Instant Pot and quick-release pressure. Carefully remove lid, allowing steam to escape away from you. 3. Discard bay leaves. Using slotted spoon, transfer onion and carrots to food processor and process until smooth, about 1 minute, scraping down sides of bowl as needed. Stir vegetable mixture into lentils and season with salt, pepper, and extra vinegar to taste. Drizzle individual portions with extra oil, and sprinkle with almonds and parsley before serving.

Per Serving

Cal: 360 | Total Fat: 16g | Sat Fat: 4.5g | Chol: 25mg | Sodium: 950mg | Total Carbs: 30g, Fiber: 7g, Total Sugar: 5g | Added Sugar: 0g | Protein: 21g

Cream of Cauliflower Gazpacho

Prep time: 15 minutes | Cook time: 25 minutes | Serves 4 to 6

- 1 cup raw almonds
- ½ cup extra-virgin olive oil, plus 1 tablespoon, divided
- 2 garlic cloves, finely minced
- 2 cups chicken or vegetable stock or broth, plus more if needed
- ½ teaspoon salt
- 1 small white onion, minced
- 1 small head cauliflower, stalk removed and broken into florets (about 3 cups)
- 1 tablespoon red wine vinegar
- ¼ teaspoon freshly ground black pepper

1. Bring a small pot of water to a boil. Add the almonds to the water and boil for 1 minute, being careful to not boil longer or the almonds will become soggy. Drain in a colander and run under cold water. Pat dry and, using your fingers, squeeze the meat of each almond out of its skin. Discard the skins. 2. In a food processor or blender, blend together the almonds and salt. With the processor running, drizzle in ½ cup extra-virgin olive oil, scraping down the sides as needed. Set the almond paste aside. 3. In a large stockpot, heat the remaining 1 tablespoon olive oil over medium-high heat. Add the onion and sauté until golden, 3 to 4 minutes. Add the cauliflower florets and sauté for another 3 to 4 minutes. Add the garlic and sauté for 1 minute more. 4. Add 2 cups stock and bring to a boil. Cover, reduce the heat to medium-low, and simmer the vegetables until tender, 8 to 10 minutes. Remove from the heat and allow to cool slightly. 5. Add the vinegar and pepper. Using an immersion blender, blend until smooth. Alternatively, you can blend in a stand blender, but you may need to divide the mixture into two or three batches. With the blender running, add the almond paste and blend until smooth, adding extra stock if the soup is too thick. 6. Serve warm, or chill in refrigerator at least 4 to 6 hours to serve a cold gazpacho.

Per Serving

Calories: 505 | Total Fat: 45g | Total Carbs: 15g | Net Carbs: 10g | Fiber: 5g | Protein: 10g | Sodium: 484mg

Lentil Sweet Potato Soup

Prep time: 15 minutes | Cook time: 30 minutes | Serves 6

- 1 tablespoon extra-virgin olive oil
- 1 carrot, diced
- 1 sweet potato, unpeeled and diced
- 1 dried bay leaf
- 1 teaspoon ground cumin
- ¼ teaspoon freshly ground black pepper
- 1 onion, diced
- 1 celery stalk, diced
- 1 cup green or brown lentils
- 1 teaspoon ground turmeric
- 1 teaspoon kosher salt
- 4 cups no-salt-added vegetable stock

1. Heat the olive oil in a large stockpot over medium-high heat. Add the onion, carrot, celery, and sweet potato and sauté 5 to 6 minutes. Add the lentils, bay leaf, turmeric, cumin, salt, and black pepper and cook for 30 seconds to 1 minute more. 2. Add the stock, bring to a boil, then lower the heat to low, and simmer, covered for 20 to 30 minutes, or until the lentils and sweet potato are tender. If you find the soup becoming thick and stew-like, feel free to add additional stock or water as it cooks.

Per Serving
Calories: 145 | Fat: 3g | Protein: 7g | Carbs: 25g | Sugars: 6g | Fiber: 7g | Sodium: 350mg | Cholesterol: 0mg

Greek Salad Soup

Prep time: 15 minutes | Cook time: 6 to 8 hours | Serves 6

- 4 tomatoes, cut into wedges
- 2 green bell peppers, seeded and diced
- 1 cup whole Kalamata olives, pitted
- 2 cups water
- 2 teaspoons red wine vinegar
- 1 teaspoon sea salt
- 4 ounces (113 g) feta cheese, crumbled
- 2 cucumbers, cut into 1-inch-thick rounds
- 1 small red onion, diced
- 4 cups low-sodium chicken broth
- 1 tablespoon extra-virgin olive oil
- 1½ teaspoons dried oregano
- ½ teaspoon freshly ground black pepper

1. In a slow cooker, combine the tomatoes, cucumbers, bell peppers, onion, olives, chicken broth, water, olive oil, vinegar, oregano, salt, and black pepper. Stir to mix well. 2. Cover the cooker and cook for 6 to 8 hours on Low heat. 3. Top each bowl with feta cheese before serving.

Per Serving
Calories: 180 | Total fat: 12g | Sodium: 976mg | Carbohydrates: 13g | Fiber: 3g | Sugar: 4g | Protein: 6g

Tuscan Bean Soup with Kale

Prep time: 20 minutes | Cook time: 25 minutes | Serves 4

- 2 tablespoons extra-virgin olive oil
- 1 carrot, diced
- 1 teaspoon kosher salt
- 1 (15 ounces / 425-g) can no-salt-added or low-sodium cannellini beans, drained and rinsed
- 1 tablespoon fresh oregano, chopped
- 1 bunch kale, stemmed and chopped
- 1 onion, diced
- 1 celery stalk, diced
- 4 cups no-salt-added vegetable stock
- 1 tablespoon fresh thyme, chopped
- 1 tablespoon fresh sage, chopped
- ¼ teaspoon freshly ground black pepper
- ¼ cup grated Parmesan cheese (optional)

1. Heat the olive oil in a large pot over medium-high heat. Add the onion, carrot, celery, and salt and sauté until translucent and slightly golden, 5 to 6 minutes. 2. Add the vegetable stock, beans, thyme, sage, oregano, and black pepper and bring to a boil. Turn down the heat to low, and simmer for 10 minutes. Stir in the kale and let it wilt, about 5 minutes. 3. Sprinkle 1 tablespoon Parmesan cheese over each bowl before serving, if desired.

Per Serving
Calories: 235 | Fat: 8g | Protein: 9g | Carbs: 35g | Sugars: 6g | Fiber: 7g | Sodium: 540mg | Cholesterol: 0mg

Cauliflower & Blue Cheese Soup

Prep time: 15 minutes | Cook time: 20 minutes | Serves 5

- 2 tablespoons (30 ml) extra-virgin avocado oil
- 1 medium (60 g/2.1 ounces / 60-g) celery stalk, sliced
- 2 cups (480 ml) vegetable or chicken stock
- ¼ cup (60 ml) goat's cream or heavy whipping cream
- 1 cup (113 g/4 ounces) crumbled goat's or sheep's blue cheese, such as Roquefort
- 1 small (60 g/2.1 ounces / 60-g) red onion, diced
- 1 medium (500 g/1.1 pounds / 499-g) cauliflower, cut into small florets
- Salt and black pepper, to taste
- 2 tablespoons (6 g/0.2 ounces) chopped fresh chives
- 5 tablespoons (75 ml) extra-virgin olive oil

1. Heat a medium saucepan greased with the avocado oil over medium heat. Sweat the onion and celery for 3 to 5 minutes, until soft and fragrant. Add the cauliflower florets and cook for 5 minutes. Add the vegetable stock and bring to a boil. Cook for about 10 minutes, or until the cauliflower is tender. Remove from the heat and let cool for a few minutes. 2. Add the cream. Use an immersion blender, or pour into a blender, to process until smooth and creamy. Season with salt and pepper to taste. Divide the soup between serving bowls and top with the crumbled blue cheese, chives, and olive oil. To store, let cool and refrigerate in a sealed container for up to 5 days.

Per Serving

Total carbs: 7.9 g | Fiber: 2.6 g | Net Carbs: 5.3 g | Protein: 7.8 g | Fat: 35.2 g (of which saturated: 12.6 g) | Calories: 372

Sicilian Fish Soup

Prep time: 20 minutes | Cook time: 33 minutes | Serves 4

- 3 tablespoons olive oil
- 1 bulb fennel, trimmed, cored, and chopped
- 2 cloves garlic, minced
- 2 cups water
- ¾ teaspoon kosher salt
- ½ pound shrimp, peeled and deveined
- ¼ cup chopped fresh flat-leaf parsley
- 1 lemon, cut into wedges
- 1 white onion, chopped
- 2 tomatoes, chopped
- ¼–½ teaspoon red-pepper flakes
- ⅔ cup dry white wine or water
- 1 pound (454 g) mussels, scrubbed and debearded
- ½ pound skin-off white fish, such as cod, halibut, or haddock, cut into 2' chunks

1. In a medium soup pot over medium heat, warm the oil. Cook the onion and fennel, stirring occasionally, until tender but not browned, 5 to 6 minutes. 2. Add the tomatoes, garlic, and pepper flakes. Cook, stirring occasionally, until the tomatoes begin to break down, 3 to 4 minutes. Add the water, wine or water, and salt and bring to a boil. Reduce the heat to a simmer and cook, stirring occasionally, to blend the flavors and soften the vegetables, about 15 minutes. 3. Add the mussels, shrimp, and fish. Cover and simmer until the shrimp and fish are cooked through and the mussels have opened (discard any that do not), 6 to 8 minutes. Stir in the parsley and serve with the lemon wedges.

Per Serving

Calories: 299 | Protein: 25g | Carbohydrates: 14g | Sugars: 3g | Total Fat: 13g | Saturated Fat: 2g | Fiber: 3g | Sodium: 948mg

Lemon Chicken Soup with Orzo

Prep time: 10 minutes | Cook time: 6 to 8 hours | Serves 6

1 pound (454 g) boneless, skinless chicken thighs or 1 pound (454 g) bone-in, skinless chicken breast
2 celery stalks, thinly sliced
1 carrot, diced
Grated zest of 1 lemon
1 bay leaf
1 teaspoon dried oregano
¾ cup dried orzo pasta
4 cups low-sodium chicken broth
2 cups water
1 small onion, diced
1 garlic clove, minced
Juice of 1 lemon
1 teaspoon sea salt
½ teaspoon freshly ground black pepper
1 lemon, thinly sliced

1. In a slow cooker, combine the chicken, chicken broth, water, celery, onion, carrot, garlic, lemon zest, lemon juice, bay leaf, salt, oregano, and pepper. Stir to mix well. 2. Cover the cooker and cook for 6 to 8 hours on Low heat. 3. Remove the chicken from the slow cooker and shred it. (If you are using bone-in chicken, remove and discard the bones while shredding. The meat should be so tender that the bones just slide out.) 4. Return the chicken to the slow cooker and add the orzo and lemon slices. 5. Replace the cover on the cooker and cook for 15 to 30 minutes on Low heat, or until the orzo is tender. 6. Remove and discard the bay leaf before serving.

Per Serving
Calories: 195 | Total fat: 5g | Sodium: 561mg | Carbohydrates: 22g | Fiber: 3g | Sugar: 2g | Protein: 15g

Saffron-Scented Chickpea Soup with Crispy Pasta

Prep time: 5 minutes | Cook time: 15 minutes | Serves 4

4 cups chicken broth
1 teaspoon salt
Pinch of saffron
2 (15 ounces / 425-g) cans chickpeas, drained and rinsed
⅓ cup olive oil
6 ounces (170 g) pappardelle or other wide ribbon-shaped pasta, cooked according to the package instructions, divided

1. In a stockpot, combine the broth and chickpeas and bring to a boil over medium-high heat. Reduce the heat to medium-low and simmer for about 5 minutes, until the chickpeas are nice and tender. Add the salt and saffron. Continue to simmer the soup over low heat. 2. Meanwhile, heat the olive oil in a large skillet over medium-high heat. Dry ⅓ of the cooked noodles well with paper towels or a clean dishtowel and add them to the hot oil. Cook, flipping as needed with a spatula, until the noodles are crisp and golden brown, about 2 minutes. Transfer the fried noodles to a paper towel-lined plate, reserving the oil in the pan. 3. Stir the remaining cooked noodles into the soup. Serve the soup hot, garnished with the fried noodles and a drizzle of the olive oil from the skillet.

Per Serving
Calories: 690 | Total Fat: 25g | Saturated Fat: 4g | Carbs: 89g | Protein: 30g | Sodium: 1,381mg | Fiber: 19g

Greek Lemon Soup with Quinoa

Prep time: 15 minutes | Cook time: 30 minutes | Serves 6 to 8

2 tablespoons olive oil
4 celery stalks, diced (generous 1 cup)
4 cups low-sodium vegetable broth
½ cup fresh lemon juice
¼ teaspoon freshly ground white pepper

1 large onion, chopped (about 2 cups)
5 carrots, diced (1 cup)
½ cup quinoa, well rinsed
3 eggs
4 cups baby kale or spinach

1. In a 3-quart saucepan, heat the olive oil over medium heat. Add the onion, celery, and carrots and sauté until translucent, about 10 minutes. Add the broth and the quinoa. Bring the broth to a boil. Reduce the heat to maintain a simmer, cover, and cook for 15 to 20 minutes, until the quinoa is cooked through. 2. In a medium bowl, beat together the lemon juice, eggs, and white pepper. While whisking, ladle 2 cups of the hot broth into the egg mixture to temper the eggs (this prevents them from scrambling from the heat of the broth). Pour the egg mixture back into the pot and stir to combine. 3. Stir in the greens and cook just until they've wilted, then serve.

Per Serving (1 cup)
Calories: 218 | Fat: 10g | Protein: 8g | Carbs: 25g | Sugars: 7g | Fiber: 5g | Sodium: 367mg | Cholesterol: 265mg

Lentil Soup with Sorrel

Prep time: 15 minutes | Cook time: 40 minutes | Serves 8

1 tablespoon olive oil
2 medium carrots, peeled and chopped (1 cup)
1 red bell pepper, seeded and chopped (1 cup)
3 garlic cloves, minced
8 cups low-sodium vegetable broth
1 bunch sorrel (or 5 ounces / 142 g baby spinach plus
1 tablespoon fresh lemon juice and ½ teaspoon lemon zest)

1 medium onion, chopped (1½ cups)
1 celery stalk, chopped (½ cup)
1 cup green or black lentils
½ teaspoon freshly ground black pepper
2 tablespoons chopped fresh parsley

1. In a stockpot, heat the olive oil over medium-high heat. Add the onion, carrots, celery, and bell pepper and sauté until the onion becomes translucent, about 10 minutes. 2. Add the lentils, garlic, and black pepper; cook for 1 minute more. Add the broth and bring to a boil. Reduce the heat to maintain a simmer and cook for 20 to 25 minutes, until the lentils are tender. 3. Stir in the parsley and sorrel; cook until wilted, 2 to 3 minutes. Serve.

Per Serving
Calories: 126 | Fat: 3g | Protein: 4g | Carbs: 21g | Sugars: 7g | Fiber: 4g | Sodium: 506mg | Cholesterol: 0mg

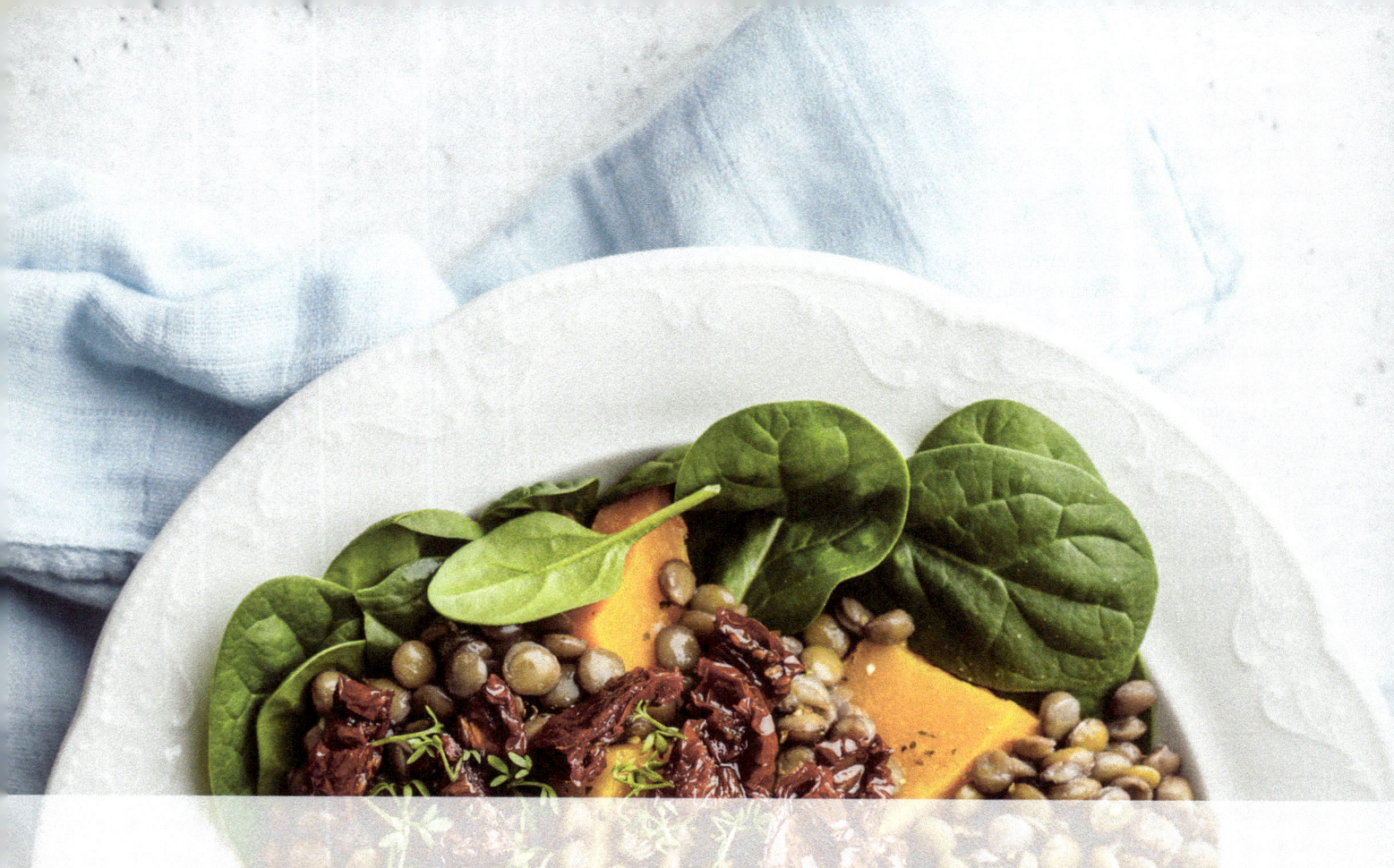

Chapter 14   Vegetables and Sides

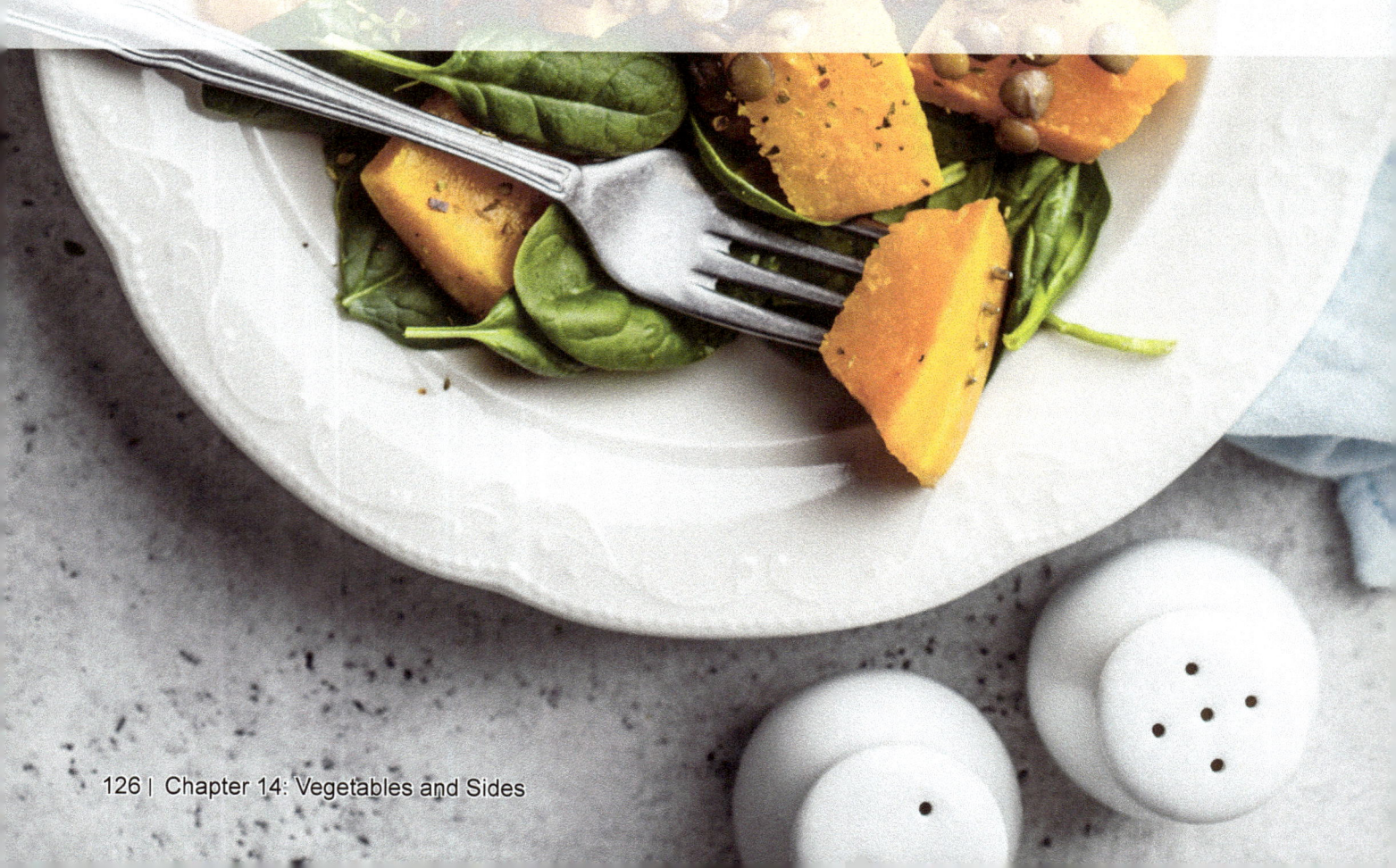

208 **Caponata (Sicilian Eggplant)** 128
209 **Vegetarian Skillet Lasagna** 128
210 **Dandelion Greens** 129
211 **Stuffed Red Peppers with Herbed Ricotta and Tomatoes** 129
212 **Sautéed Fava Beans with Olive Oil, Garlic, and Chiles** 129
213 **Puff Pastry Turnover with Roasted Vegetables** 130
214 **Puréed Cauliflower Soup** 130
215 **Roasted Brussels Sprouts with Tahini-Yogurt Sauce** 130
216 **Eggplant Caponata** 131
217 **Braised Fennel with radicchio, Pear, and Pecorino** 131
218 **Mediterranean Cauliflower Tabbouleh** 132
219 **Herb Vinaigrette Potato Salad** 132
220 **White Beans with Tomatoes, Kale, and Pancetta** 133
221 **Walnut and Freekeh Pilaf** 133

Caponata (Sicilian Eggplant)

Prep time: 1 hour 5 minutes | Cook time: 40 minutes | Serves 2

3 medium eggplant, cut into ½-inch (1.25cm) cubes (about 1.5pounds/680g)
1 medium onion (red or white), chopped
½ cup green olives, pitted and halved
3 medium tomatoes (about 15ounces/425g), chopped
2 tablespoons granulated sugar
Freshly ground black pepper to taste
1 tablespoon toasted pine nuts (optional)
½ teaspoons fine sea salt
¼ cup extra virgin olive oil
1 tablespoon dried oregano
2 tablespoons capers, rinsed
3 tablespoons red wine vinegar
Salt to taste
2 tablespoons chopped fresh basil

1. Place the eggplant in a large colander. Sprinkle ½ teaspoon sea salt over the top and set the eggplant aside to rest for about an hour. 2. Add the olive oil to a large pan over medium heat. When the oil starts to shimmer, add the eggplant and sauté until it starts to turn golden brown, about 5 minutes. Add the onions and continue sautéing until the onions become soft. 3. Add the oregano, olives, capers, and tomatoes (with juices) to the pan. Reduce the heat to medium-low and simmer for about 20–25 minutes. 4. While the onions and tomatoes are cooking, combine the vinegar and sugar in a small bowl. Stir until the sugar is completely dissolved, then add the mixture to the pan. Continue cooking for 2–3 more minutes or until you can no longer smell the vinegar and then remove the pan from the heat. 5. Season the mixture to taste with salt and black pepper. Just prior to serving, top each serving with a sprinkle of chopped basil and toasted pine nuts, if using. Store in the refrigerator for up to 3 days.

Per Serving
Calories: 235 | Total fat: 16g | Saturated fat: 2g | Carbohydrate: 20g | Protein: 3g

Vegetarian Skillet Lasagna

Prep time: 20 minutes | Cook time: 45 minutes | Serves 4

15 ounces (425 g) ricotta cheese
¼ teaspoon Italian seasoning
1 onion, coarsely chopped
2 yellow squash, quartered lengthwise and sliced into 1-inch pieces
1 carrot, cut into long ribbons
1 (28 ounces / 794 g) can crushed tomatoes
Sea salt
9 no-bake lasagna noodles, broken into 2-inch pieces
½ cup shredded mozzarella cheese
¼ cup chopped fresh Italian parsley
3 tablespoons olive oil
3 garlic cloves, minced
8 ounces (227 g) cremini (baby bella) mushrooms, quartered
6 ounces (170 g) baby spinach
1½ cups heavy (whipping) cream
Freshly ground black pepper
1 cup grated Parmesan cheese

1. Preheat the oven to 375°F (191°C). 2. In a medium bowl, stir together the ricotta, parsley, and Italian seasoning and set aside. 3. In a large oven-safe skillet, heat the olive oil over medium-high heat. Add the onion and garlic and sauté for 3 minutes. Add the squash and sauté for 2 minutes more. Add the mushrooms and sauté for 4 minutes. Add the carrot and spinach and sauté for 1 minute. 4. Add the crushed tomatoes and the cream and season with salt and pepper. Add the lasagna noodles and mix well, making sure all the noodles are entirely covered with the sauce. Dollop the ricotta mixture evenly over the tomato mixture, using the back of a spoon to gently spread it around. Evenly top with the Parmesan and mozzarella. Cover the skillet with a lid and transfer it to the oven. Bake for 20 minutes, then remove the lid and bake for 10 to 15 minutes more, until the cheese is golden brown. 5. Remove from the oven and serve.

Per Serving
Calories: 1,026 | Total fat: 69g | Total carbs: 71g | Sugar: 21g | Protein: 37g | Fiber: 9g | Sodium: 933mg

Dandelion Greens

Prep time: 10 minutes | Cook time: 1 minute | Serves 6

- 4 pounds (1.8 kg) dandelion greens, stalks cut and discarded, and greens washed
- ¼ cup lemon juice
- ½ teaspoon ground black pepper
- ½ cup water
- ¼ cup extra-virgin olive oil
- ½ teaspoon salt

1. Add dandelion greens and water to the Instant Pot®. Close lid, set steam release to Sealing, press the Manual button, and set time to 1 minute. When the timer beeps, quick-release the pressure until the float valve drops. Open lid and drain well. 2. Combine olive oil, lemon juice, salt, and pepper in a small bowl. Pour over greens and toss to coat.

Per Serving
Calories: 39 | Fat: 12g | Protein: 1g | Sodium: 253mg | Fiber: 3 | Carbohydrates: 7g | Sugar: 0g

Stuffed Red Peppers with Herbed Ricotta and Tomatoes

Prep time: 10 minutes | Cook time: 20 minutes | Serves 4

- 2 red bell peppers
- 2 Roma tomatoes, diced
- ¼ teaspoon salt
- 4 ounces (113 g) ricotta
- 3 tablespoons fresh oregano, chopped
- 1 cup cooked brown rice
- 1 garlic clove, minced
- ¼ teaspoon black pepper
- 3 tablespoons fresh basil, chopped
- ¼ cup shredded Parmesan, for topping

1. Preheat the air fryer to 360°F (182°C). 2. Cut the bell peppers in half and remove the seeds and stem. 3. In a medium bowl, combine the brown rice, tomatoes, garlic, salt, and pepper. 4. Distribute the rice filling evenly among the four bell pepper halves. 5. In a small bowl, combine the ricotta, basil, and oregano. Put the herbed cheese over the top of the rice mixture in each bell pepper. 6. Place the bell peppers into the air fryer and roast for 20 minutes. 7. Remove and serve with shredded Parmesan on top.

Per Serving
Calories: 156 | Total Fat: 6g | Saturated Fat: 3g | Protein: 8g | Total Carbohydrates: 19g | Fiber: 3g | Sugar: 4g | Cholesterol: 18mg

Sautéed Fava Beans with Olive Oil, Garlic, and Chiles

Prep time: 10 minutes | Cook time: 7 minutes | Serves 4

- 3½ pounds (1.6kg) fresh fava beans, shelled (4 cups)
- 2 cloves garlic, minced
- 1 teaspoon finely grated lemon zest
- ½ teaspoon salt
- 2 tablespoons olive oil
- 2 teaspoons fresh lemon juice
- ½ teaspoon crushed red pepper flakes
- ¼ teaspoon freshly ground black pepper

1. Bring a medium saucepan of lightly salted water to a boil. Add the shelled favas and cook for 3 to 4 minutes, until tender. Drain the favas and immediately place them in an ice water bath to stop their cooking. When cool, peel the tough outer skin off the beans. 2. Heat the olive oil in a large skillet over medium-high heat. Add the garlic and cook, stirring, until it is aromatic but not browned, about 30 seconds. Add the beans and cook, stirring, until heated through, about 2 minutes. Stir in the lemon juice, lemon zest, red pepper flakes, salt, and pepper and remove from the heat. Serve immediately.

Per Serving
Calories: 576 | Total Fat: 9g | Saturated Fat: 1g | Carbs: 88g | Protein: 39g | Sodium: 311mg | Fiber: 38g

Puff Pastry Turnover with Roasted Vegetables

Prep time: 10 minutes | Cook time: 35 minutes | Serves 4 to 6

Nonstick cooking spray
½ bunch asparagus, cut into quarters
1 large egg, beaten
1 zucchini, cut in ¼-inch-thick slices
1 package (6-inch) whole-grain pastry discs, in the freezer section (Goya brand preferred), at room temperature

1. Preheat the oven to 350°F (177°C). 2. Spray a baking sheet with cooking spray and arrange the zucchini and asparagus on it in a single layer. Roast for 15 to 20 minutes, until tender. Set aside to cool. 3. Allow the pastry dough to warm to room temperature. Place the discs on a floured surface. 4. Place a roasted zucchini slice on one half of each disc, then top with asparagus. Fold the empty side over the full side and pinch the turnover closed with a fork. 5. Once all discs are full and closed, brush the turnovers with the beaten egg and put them onto a baking sheet. Bake for 10 to 15 minutes, until golden brown. Let cool completely before eating.

Per Serving
Calories: 334 | Protein: 9g | Total Carbohydrates: 42g | Sugars: 3g | Fiber: 4g | Total Fat: 15g | Saturated Fat: 8g | Cholesterol: 47mg | Sodium: 741mg

Puréed Cauliflower Soup

Prep time: 15 minutes | Cook time: 11 minutes | Serves 6

2 tablespoons olive oil
1 stalk celery, chopped
3 sprigs fresh thyme
2 cups vegetable stock
¼ cup low-fat plain Greek yogurt
1 medium onion, peeled and chopped
1 medium carrot, peeled and chopped
4 cups cauliflower florets
½ cup half-and-half
2 tablespoons chopped fresh chives

1. Press the Sauté button on the Instant Pot® and heat oil. Add onion, celery, and carrot. Cook until just tender, about 6 minutes. Add thyme, cauliflower, and stock. Stir well, then press the Cancel button. 2. Close lid, set steam release to Sealing, press the Manual button, and set time to 5 minutes. When the timer beeps, let pressure release naturally, about 15 minutes. 3. Open lid, remove and discard thyme stems, and with an immersion blender, purée soup until smooth. Stir in half-and-half and yogurt. Garnish with chives and serve immediately.

Per Serving
Calories: 113 | Fat: 7g | Protein: 3g | Sodium: 236mg | Fiber: 2 | Carbohydrates: 9g | Sugar: 5g

Roasted Brussels Sprouts with Tahini-Yogurt Sauce

Prep time: 10 minutes | Cook time: 35 minutes | Serves 4

1 pound (454 g) Brussels sprouts, trimmed and halved lengthwise
½ teaspoon garlic powder
¼ cup plain whole-milk Greek yogurt
Zest and juice of 1 lemon
6 tablespoons extra-virgin olive oil, divided
1 teaspoon salt, divided
¼ teaspoon freshly ground black pepper
¼ cup tahini

1. Preheat the oven to 425°F (218°C). Line a baking sheet with aluminum foil or parchment paper and set aside. 2. Place the Brussels sprouts in a large bowl. Drizzle with 4 tablespoons olive oil, ½ teaspoon salt, the garlic powder, and pepper and toss well to coat. 3. Place the Brussels sprouts in a single layer on the baking sheet, reserving the bowl, and roast for 20 minutes. Remove from the oven and give the sprouts a toss to flip. Return to the oven and continue to roast until browned and crispy, another 10 to 15 minutes. Remove from the oven and return to the reserved bowl. 4. In a small bowl, whisk together the yogurt, tahini, lemon zest and juice, remaining 2 tablespoons olive oil, and remaining ½ teaspoon salt. Drizzle over the roasted sprouts and toss to coat. Serve warm.

Per Serving
Calories: 358 | Total Fat: 30g | Total Carbs: 15g | Net Carbs: 9g | Fiber: 6g | Protein: 7g | Sodium: 636mg

Eggplant Caponata

Prep time: 20 minutes | Cook time: 5 minutes | Serves 8

- ¼ cup extra-virgin olive oil
- 2 tablespoons red wine vinegar
- 1 large eggplant, peeled and diced
- 1 medium green bell pepper, seeded and diced
- 2 cloves garlic, peeled and minced
- 3 stalks celery, diced
- ½ cup golden raisins
- ½ teaspoon salt
- ¼ cup white wine
- 1 teaspoon ground cinnamon
- 1 medium onion, peeled and diced
- 1 medium red bell pepper, seeded and diced
- 1 (14½ ounces / 411 g) can diced tomatoes
- ½ cup chopped oil-cured olives
- 2 tablespoons capers, rinsed and drained
- ½ teaspoon ground black pepper

1. Place all ingredients in the Instant Pot®. Stir well to mix. Close lid, set steam release to Sealing, press the Manual button, and set time to 5 minutes. 2. When the timer beeps, quick-release the pressure until the float valve drops.
Open the lid and stir well. Serve warm or at room temperature.

Per Serving
Calories: 90 | Fat: 1g | Protein: 2g | Sodium: 295mg | Fiber: 4 | Carbohydrates: 17g | Sugar: 13g

Braised Fennel with radicchio, Pear, and Pecorino

Prep time: 20 minutes | Cook time: 12 minutes | Serves 4

- 6 tablespoons extra-virgin olive oil, divided
- ¾ teaspoon table salt, divided
- ½ teaspoon grated lemon zest plus 4 teaspoons juice
- 5 ounces / 142-g (5 cups) baby arugula
- 1 Bosc or Bartlett pear, quartered, cored, and sliced thin
- 2 fennel bulbs (12 ounces each), 2 tablespoons fronds chopped, stalks discarded, bulbs halved, each half cut into 1-inch-thick wedges
- 1 small head radicchio (5 ounces / 170 g), shredded
- ¼ cup whole almonds, toasted and chopped
- Shaved Pecorino Romano cheese

1. Using highest sauté function, heat 2 tablespoons oil in Instant Pot for 5 minutes (or until just smoking). Brown half of fennel, about 3 minutes per side; transfer to plate. Repeat with 1 tablespoon oil and remaining fennel; do not remove from pot. 2. Return first batch of fennel to pot along with ½ cup water and ½ teaspoon salt. Lock lid in place and close pressure release valve. Select high pressure cook function and cook for 2 minutes. Turn off Instant Pot and quick-release pressure. Carefully remove lid, allowing steam to escape away from you. Using slotted spoon, transfer fennel to plate; discard cooking liquid. 3. Whisk remaining 3 tablespoons oil, lemon zest and juice, and remaining ¼ teaspoon salt together in large bowl. Add arugula, radicchio, and pear and toss to coat. Transfer arugula mixture to serving dish and arrange fennel wedges on top. Sprinkle with almonds, fennel fronds, and Pecorino. Serve.

Per Serving
Cal: 290 | Total Fat: 26g | Sat Fat: 3.5g | Chol: 0mg | Sodium: 300mg | Total Carbs: 22g, Fiber: 7g, Total Sugar: 11g | Added Sugar: 0g | Protein: 5g

Mediterranean Cauliflower Tabbouleh

Prep time: 15 minutes | Cook time: 5 minutes | Serves 6

6 tablespoons extra-virgin olive oil, divided
3 garlic cloves, finely minced
½ teaspoon freshly ground black pepper
½ cup chopped mint leaves
½ cup chopped pitted Kalamata olives
Juice of 1 lemon (about 2 tablespoons)
2 medium avocados, peeled, pitted, and diced
4 cups riced cauliflower
1½ teaspoons salt
½ large cucumber, peeled, seeded, and chopped
½ cup chopped Italian parsley
2 tablespoons minced red onion
2 cups baby arugula or spinach leaves
1 cup quartered cherry tomatoes

1. In a large skillet, heat 2 tablespoons of olive oil over medium-high heat. Add the riced cauliflower, garlic, salt, and pepper and sauté until just tender but not mushy, 3 to 4 minutes. Remove from the heat and place in a large bowl. 2. Add the cucumber, mint, parsley, olives, red onion, lemon juice, and remaining 4 tablespoons olive oil and toss well. Place in the refrigerator, uncovered, and refrigerate for at least 30 minutes, or up to 2 hours. 3. Before serving, add the arugula, avocado, and tomatoes and toss to combine well. Season to taste with salt and pepper and serve cold or at room temperature.

Per Serving
Calories: 235 | Total Fat: 21g | Total Carbs: 12g | Net Carbs: 6g | Fiber: 6g | Protein: 4g | Sodium: 623mg

Herb Vinaigrette Potato Salad

Prep time: 10 minutes | Cook time: 4 minutes | Serves 10

¼ cup olive oil
¼ cup chopped fresh flat-leaf parsley
2 tablespoons chopped fresh chives
½ teaspoon dry mustard powder
2 pounds (907g) baby Yukon Gold potatoes
1 teaspoon salt
3 tablespoons red wine vinegar
2 tablespoons chopped fresh dill
1 clove garlic, peeled and minced
¼ teaspoon ground black pepper
1 cup water

1. Whisk together oil, vinegar, parsley, dill, chives, garlic, mustard, and pepper in a small bowl. Set aside. 2. Place potatoes in a steamer basket. Place the rack in the Instant Pot®, add water and salt, then top with the steamer basket. Close lid, set steam release to Sealing, press the Manual button, and set time to 4 minutes. When the timer beeps, quick-release the pressure until the float valve drops. Press the Cancel button and open lid. 3. Transfer hot potatoes to a serving bowl. Pour dressing over potatoes and gently toss to coat. Serve warm or at room temperature.

Per Serving
Calories: 116 | Fat: 6g | Protein: 2g | Sodium: 239mg | Fiber: 1 | Carbohydrates: 16g | Sugar: 1g

White Beans with Tomatoes, Kale, and Pancetta

Prep time: 5 minutes | Cook time: 20 minutes | Serves 4

1 tablespoon olive oil
1 pound (454 g) kale, tough center ribs removed, leaves julienned
2 dried hot red chiles
1 teaspoon finely chopped rosemary
1 (15 ounces / 425-g) can diced tomatoes with juice
Freshly ground black pepper
4 ounces (113 g) pancetta, diced
1 medium onion, diced
2 cloves garlic, thinly sliced
¾ teaspoon salt
1 teaspoon finely chopped sage
1 (19 ounces) can cannellini beans, drained and rinsed

1. Heat the olive oil in a large skillet over medium-high heat. Add the pancetta and cook, stirring frequently, until the fat begins to render, about 3 minutes. Reduce the heat to medium, add the kale, onion, garlic, chiles, and salt, and cook, stirring frequently, until the onion is softened and beginning to brown, about 7 minutes. Stir in the rosemary and sage and then the tomatoes along with their juice. Bring to a simmer. 2. Stir in the beans to the skillet and cook, stirring occasionally, until the sauce begins to thicken, about 7 more minutes. Taste and add pepper if needed. Serve hot.

Per Serving
Calories: 722 | Total Fat: 17g | Saturated Fat: 5g | Carbs: 101g | Protein: 47g | Sodium: 1,181mg | Fiber: 37g

Walnut and Freekeh Pilaf

Prep time: 15 minutes | Cook time: 15 minutes | Serves 4

2½ cups freekeh
2 medium onions, diced
¼ teaspoon ground allspice
½ cup chopped walnuts
Freshly ground black pepper
1½ teaspoons freshly squeezed lemon juice
3 tablespoons extra-virgin olive oil, divided
¼ teaspoon ground cinnamon
5 cups chicken stock
Salt
½ cup plain, unsweetened, full-fat Greek yogurt
½ teaspoon garlic powder

1. In a small bowl, soak the freekeh covered in cold water for 5 minutes. Drain and rinse the freekeh, then rinse one more time. 2. In a large sauté pan or skillet, heat 2 tablespoons oil, then add the onions and cook until fragrant. Add the freekeh, cinnamon, and allspice. Stir periodically for 1 minute. 3. Add the stock and walnuts and season with salt and pepper. Bring to a simmer. 4. Cover and reduce the heat to low. Cook for 15 minutes. Once freekeh is tender, remove from the heat and allow to rest for 5 minutes. 5. In a small bowl, combine the yogurt, lemon juice, and garlic powder. You may need to add salt to bring out the flavors. Add the yogurt mixture to the freekeh and serve immediately.

Per Serving
Calories: 653 | Protein: 23g | Total Carbohydrates: 91g | Sugars: 4g | Fiber: 12g | Total Fat: 25g | Saturated Fat: 3g | Cholesterol: 4mg | Sodium: 575mg

Appendix 1 Measurement Conversion Chart

VOLUME EQUIVALENTS(DRY)

US STANDARD	METRIC (APPROXIMATE)
1/8 teaspoon	0.5 mL
1/4 teaspoon	1 mL
1/2 teaspoon	2 mL
3/4 teaspoon	4 mL
1 teaspoon	5 mL
1 tablespoon	15 mL
1/4 cup	59 mL
1/2 cup	118 mL
3/4 cup	177 mL
1 cup	235 mL
2 cups	475 mL
3 cups	700 mL
4 cups	1 L

VOLUME EQUIVALENTS(LIQUID)

US STANDARD	US STANDARD (OUNCES)	METRIC (APPROXIMATE)
2 tablespoons	1 fl.oz.	30 mL
1/4 cup	2 fl.oz.	60 mL
1/2 cup	4 fl.oz.	120 mL
1 cup	8 fl.oz.	240 mL
1 1/2 cup	12 fl.oz.	355 mL
2 cups or 1 pint	16 fl.oz.	475 mL
4 cups or 1 quart	32 fl.oz.	1 L
1 gallon	128 fl.oz.	4 L

WEIGHT EQUIVALENTS

US STANDARD	METRIC (APPROXIMATE)
1 ounce	28 g
2 ounces	57 g
5 ounces	142 g
10 ounces	284 g
15 ounces	425 g
16 ounces (1 pound)	455 g
1.5 pounds	680 g
2 pounds	907 g

TEMPERATURES EQUIVALENTS

FAHRENHEIT(F)	CELSIUS(C) (APPROXIMATE)
225 °F	107 °C
250 °F	120 °C
275 °F	135 °C
300 °F	150 °C
325 °F	160 °C
350 °F	180 °C
375 °F	190 °C
400 °F	205 °C
425 °F	220 °C
450 °F	235 °C
475 °F	245 °C
500 °F	260 °C

Appendix 2 The Dirty Dozen and Clean Fifteen

The Environmental Working Group (EWG) is a nonprofit, nonpartisan organization dedicated to protecting human health and the environment Its mission is to empower people to live healthier lives in a healthier environment. This organization publishes an annual list of the twelve kinds of produce, in sequence, that have the highest amount of pesticide residue-the Dirty Dozen-as well as a list of the fifteen kinds of produce that have the least amount of pesticide residue-the Clean Fifteen.

THE DIRTY DOZEN

- The 2016 Dirty Dozen includes the following produce. These are considered among the year's most important produce to buy organic:

Strawberries	Spinach
Apples	Tomatoes
Nectarines	Bell peppers
Peaches	Cherry tomatoes
Celery	Cucumbers
Grapes	Kale/collard greens
Cherries	Hot peppers

- The Dirty Dozen list contains two additional items kale/collard greens and hot peppers-because they tend to contain trace levels of highly hazardous pesticides.

THE CLEAN FIFTEEN

- The least critical to buy organically are the Clean Fifteen list. The following are on the 2016 list:

Avocados	Papayas
Corn	Kiw
Pineapples	Eggplant
Cabbage	Honeydew
Sweet peas	Grapefruit
Onions	Cantaloupe
Asparagus	Cauliflower
Mangos	

- Some of the sweet corn sold in the United States are made from genetically engineered (GE) seedstock. Buy organic varieties of these crops to avoid GE produce.